Praise for SCOTT HARLOW

"Scott Harlow is focused, goal driven and never quits."
— **BRAD MCLEOD,** *Retired Navy* SEAL *and CEO of* SEAL GRINDER PT

"Scott gave me the ability to consider my absolute maximum effort to be nothing more than a starting point."
— **LAURA STEWART,** *Physical Therapist,* PCT *Thru Hiker*

"Scott's *mindset* is his superpower. He drives, he leads, but most importantly…he just doesn't quit."
— **PAUL LAMOUREUX,** *Master of Arts in Leadership, Certified Executive Coach, and Former Emergency Response Team Sniper*

"He who has a why to live for can bear with almost any how"

— VIKTOR FRANKL

DO IT ANYWAY

OVERCOME YOUR PERCEIVED PHYSICAL AND MENTAL LIMITS

SCOTT HARLOW

Above the Noise

To my brother Mark. You are always with me.

© 2021 Scott Harlow. All rights reserved.

No part of this book may be used or reproduced in any manner whatsoever without the express written permission of the publisher or author. The exception would be in the case of brief quotations embodied in critical articles or reviews, and pages where permission is specifically granted by the publisher or author, or in the case of photocopying, a licence from Access Copyright, www.accesscopyright.ca, 1-800-893-5777, info@accesscopyright.ca.

Library of Canada Cataloguing in Publication data is available.

ISBN 978-1-989528-06-8 (paperback edition)

ISBN 978-1-989528-07-5 (e-book edition)

First Edition Printing 2021

Front cover photo by Derek Ford

Book design by Clint Hutzulak

Edited by Susheela Kundargi & Sofia Del Carmen Capel

'Before' photo courtesy of the author; 'after' photo by Shawn Aylesworth

Published in Canada by Above the Noise, New Glasgow, NS
www.abovethenoisepublishing.com.

For more information contact: publishing@abovethenoise.ca

Special discounts are available on quantity purchases by corporations, associations, and others. For details, contact the publisher at the address above.

For more information on the book and author please visit www.scottharlow.ca

CONTENTS

Introduction   1

Part 1

Chapter 1	Alberta	9
Chapter 2	Hockey	15
Chapter 3	Modeling	25
Chapter 4	Car Sales	33
Chapter 5	Divine Intervention	39
Chapter 6	Turning Point	49

Part 2

Chapter 7	Kokoro 44, First 24 hours	59
Chapter 8	Kokoro 44, Second Night	73
Chapter 9	Kokoro 51	85
Chapter 10	GORUCK Selection 021, Part 1	105
Chapter 11	GORUCK Selection 021, Part 2	129
Chapter 12	Things I've Learned	139
Chapter 13	Do It Anyway!	151

Epilogue   157
Acknowledgements   161
About the Author   163

INTRODUCTION

Beach Workout
Ruck on
30 Hydro burpees
50 m bear crawl
20 Hydro burpees
50 m walking lunge
10 Hydro burpees
50 m OH carry
20 Hydro burpees
50 m low crawl
30 Hydro burpees
50 m sandbag toss

It is four o'clock in the morning and I am standing with a 60-pound backpack on next to a Florida swamp, drenched in my own sweat and urine. The mud and sand cemented between my body and the pack has chafed away every bit of skin it has rubbed against, my groin is raw and bleeding from what feels like sandpaper wedged between my legs. "I quit." There is no taking it back. "I QUIT" — The words spill over my lips like many times before. I throw my rucksack on the ground and walk over to the truck. It is like watching myself from the side-lines as I limp up to the vehicle. "Hey, Cadre Mocha Mike, I'm done!"

"Why? You look strong."

"I'm not putting that fucking ruck back on."

Mike looks at me and says "Okay" and with those words I'm out. Once the words are spoken it is final. There is no taking it back.

It is October 18, 2019, I am fifty-three years old, quitting once again.

With its forty-eight-plus hours, eighty-plus miles, and an average pass rate of less than two percent, GORUCK Selection is considered the toughest endurance event in the world. Patterned directly after Special Forces Selection, the cadre actively try to make you quit. Their role is to methodically enforce a standard very few people in the world can achieve, and you are performance dropped if you fail to meet the standard. You are pushed well beyond what you ever thought capable of. Many are pushed too far. In my case, I quit as the sixteenth participant left in the event, down from the 224 that had signed up and fifty-nine that showed. After I quit, I sugarcoated the situation by saying: "I tapped out." But upon reflection, while sitting beside the swamp, engulfed in the cold, chafing and miserable, it seeps into my mind; there is no denying I had quit.

I am no stranger to quitting and have done it many times before; when the going got tough, when I lacked confidence or when my arrogance got the better of me. Quitting is sometimes necessary; when some vices became life-threatening, I quit those too. But quitting this time was different.

I didn't need to tell anyone I had quit; the event was broadcast live and those watching knew I was done. Before calling friends and family back home I gave it a day. People love to tell you what they think you want to hear.

"You made it further than most. Congratulations."

"You should be proud of your achievement!"

But I know that, with everything I have accomplished, the self-imposed limits I've ploughed through, how much I've changed: It doesn't matter how far I made it, I simply didn't finish.

When describing the details of this grueling event, most say, "Of course you quit! That event is insane!" But I am not looking for an excuse to feel good about giving up. I'm looking for fuel to keep going.

I hadn't quit on a whim, simply to follow the next big thing. I didn't quit because I could no longer sit back on what came easily to me, nor was I just mildly uncomfortable; I had transformed from that quitter. I knew exactly what changes needed to occur in order to succeed or at least give me the best chances of succeeding the next time.

With hard work, I have reached a high level of mental toughness and peak physical form. From my own journey, I know the following to be true: if I can do it, so can you. There's absolutely nothing special, genetically different or better about me. I wish I had a superpower to make me unstoppable, but I don't. I've just busted my ass to overcome physical and mental obstacles.

If you don't have a "WHY," attempting an extreme endurance event is useless. When things get difficult, it's your "WHY" that carries you through to the end. And if the "WHY" isn't big enough, you'll quit.

Having a "WHY" is crucial for getting through difficult times. Going into Selection my "WHY" was to be an example to people over forty that you can push your body to the limit and do things beyond your imagination. I want to inspire people to get off of the couch and take control of their health and fitness. This is the reason for "Do it anyway".

Ruck and Sandbag PT
50 lb Ruck
82 lb Sand bag
Warm up - 400 m run
3 rounds - 30 SS
15 squats
10 push ups

Ruck on for duration
100 m Bear crawl
100 m low crawl
50 m crab walk
50 m duck walk
100 m overhead lunge
100 m sandbag clean and throw
50 m low crawl sandbag drag
50 m OH carry

Huge Suck factor

CHAPTER 1

ALBERTA

I was born in Drumheller, Alberta, Canada in November, 1965. It was a quaint but sleepy Badlands town surrounded by many similar little towns, about ninety minutes northeast of Calgary. My father was an RCMP (Royal Canadian Mounted Police) officer and we were transferred to different locations in Alberta for the majority of my formative years. Much like the military. Before my tenth birthday, my little brothers and I had witnessed all of our furniture, trunks of clothes and boxes of toys lifted in and out of moving trucks more times than we cared to count. We spent a few months in the new house, sometimes a year or two, and then the movers reappeared on our street and we were uprooted once more. While other boys my age formed relationships that would last a lifetime, I went from school to school with no one to call my best friend. As soon as I made a buddy or two, it was time to move again. When we finally settled in Edmonton in the mid-1970s I had become a shy and insecure kid, unsure of where and how I fit in.

I had changed schools in the middle of the sixth grade. Despite my teacher's best efforts to pair me with the class clown, I remained an outcast. As if being the new kid wasn't bad enough, I somehow managed to flip my status as the shy kid to being seen as a total boaster with just one sentence. This was during the early years of the Canada Fitness Award Program — a nation-wide competition where school kids were tested to measure their physical capabilities. The different components were running, flexed arm hangs, shuttle run, speed sit-ups, and the standing long jump. The most successful kids were awarded medals of bronze, silver or gold, preceded by the most prestigious prize: The *Award of Excellence*. The latter was only obtained on rare occasions, but somehow I had managed to get it two years in a row.

"No one here has ever won the award of excellence," stated a kid in my new school.

"Well, I have two," I proudly proclaimed, and watched as the kid's eyes turned, not green with envy, but black with rage. Nobody believed me and I ran home from school that day. The next day I proudly brought in the badges, deepening the other kids' anger, the opposite effect of what I had hoped for.

During the years to come, I continued to walk around the school like a ghost. I held my head down and kept a low profile. The in-kids shunned me. Today I wonder if it was due to jealousy. I was tall and athletically built, maybe that intimidated some of the other students. I remember walking through the halls and seeing a group of them. Their heads turned as I passed them. Someone dropped a nasty comment and as I turned around they started sniggering and pretended not to see me, as if I had imagined it all. The words hit me like daggers. They were only uttered in big groups, making it impossible for me to know who had said it. It was a form of gaslighting; a "mindfuck" that made me doubt myself even more.

I did have one friend, Jamie, who lived next door. At the end of each day I would run home and hang out with him. Till this day, he remains my closest friend. But I would not associate with the kids at school whatsoever. Looking back, it could have just been an excuse, another reason to withdraw. If this had happened today, I could easily tell them where to go. Fortunately, there's a big difference in how we see the world as adults. But as a kid, I didn't have the coping mechanisms to deal with it. I didn't even have the courage to tell my parents.

There were many instances in my childhood that contributed to, and reinforced, my feelings of shame and fear. I remember having to get up in front of the classroom in the second grade, to give a presentation about frogs. As I fumbled with the handwritten notes some of the other kids started sighing loudly and as I began talking, one shouted "boring!"

Despite the teacher's best attempts to hush the class, the circus was already in full swing. The boys riled each other up, made fart noises and the girls giggled hysterically. To this day I still fight the fear when having to speak publicly.

I started acting just a year ago and auditioning utterly terrifies me. Every time I'm in front of a casting director I am taken back to that classroom, feeling vulnerable and scared. But I do it anyway. Even if I'm terrified, I get up there, I do the job to the best of my ability. I was recently cast in a play, hoping it will help overcome any fear of auditioning and public speaking. Needless to say, I am scared shitless.

However, as a child, as many young boys did, I used sports as a vessel to be accepted by my peers. Luckily, I had some skill, especially when it came to hockey. My physique helped me establish my presence on the team which was ultimately the extent of my social circle. I didn't have many friends and any of the groups that I wanted to belong to, didn't want me.

But sports saved me. The rink was the one place where, no matter how quirky, weird, or unacceptable I might have felt in everyday life, in school or among friends, I was accepted due to my contributions. Most of the guys that I played hockey with went to other schools. All the off-ice shyness didn't diminish my on-ice performance whatsoever and often made me work harder.

We practised or played daily, and when I played Jr. hockey, it was twice per day. We usually practised in the morning and played a game at night. I don't know what it's like for kids in the rest of the country, but competitive hockey in Alberta was a daily thing.

In addition to that, there was the off-ice training. My dad had me lifting weights and running hills, preparing during the off-season. My parents allowed me to have my own goals though and were always supportive by not putting undo pressure on me to succeed in sports. I put enough pressure on myself for everyone. They were really wonderful in that way. My dad went to every game, practice or whatever sport-related activity I was involved in. He would even show up in his police car, in uniform to watch me play. It was my dream as a kid to play in the NHL. That was just all there was to it; nothing was going to stop me. Except for myself.

> *Afraid to share your fears?* "Do it anyway!"

CHAPTER 2

HOCKEY

I'm lying on a stretcher in a speeding ambulance with my dad sitting next to me. I can't see him; I can only hear his words of encouragement as he chokes back the tears. My face, or what is left of it, pulsates and all I can think is: Screw you, God. How could you let this happen to me?

As a teenager, my mind was constantly on hockey. My younger brothers, Mark and Todd, played too, but while I played competitively, they just played for fun. I didn't spend much time with them. They usually did their own thing together, and I was off doing mine; playing hockey all the time and hanging out with the kids my age. I was just over two years older than Mark, who was eighteen months older than Todd. They were the best of friends, but to me, they were just annoying little kids. In hindsight, I wish I could go back in time and appreciate them for what they were: My own flesh and blood, my protectees and later on, the best link to my past. When we were all at home, however, we did play ping pong and hand hockey in the basement, but that was the extent of it. By the time I was sixteen years old, I was off to play hockey in the SJHL (Saskatchewan Junior Hockey League).

I had played in the SJHL for a year when I decided that the next step on the road to the NHL was to play in the WHL (Western Hockey League), but no one had scouted me. When an expansion team, the Kelowna Wings, came into the league, I took matters into my own hands and sent them a letter. I asked them for a try-out, and to my delight, they said yes.

The try-out was held in Revelstoke, British Columbia. The moment I stepped onto the ice, the shy and awkward seventeen-year-old transformed. Anywhere else I did my best to stay hidden and unseen, but on the ice, I lit it up. I scored one goal after another, and for every goal, I levitated.

During an interview with the local Kelowna newspaper, our coach mentioned a player who had seemingly come out of nowhere to earn a spot on the team. How excited they were to have him and how he had a really bright future. While reading, it slowly dawned on me: that guy was me! I had to read my name several times for it to register. I had made it! Triumphantly, I put the paper down and leaned back on the couch. My body relaxed, knowing that I had done enough. The coach approved of me, and that was all I needed, right? And that is when I immediately stopped trying. This was a life-long pattern of doing just enough to make it; I thought I was at the top of the mountain when really I had only just made it to base camp. I had made the team and now I had all the confidence in the world that I wouldn't need to work hard to stay on the team. It didn't last long.

With good reason, the coach was furious at my lack of effort and I pleaded, "Just give me another chance." He said, "No. You're traded to New West". I packed up my car in silence and drove to New Westminster. By the time I started playing for the new team, I felt completely deflated. Normally when entering the rink, the familiar smells and rush of adrenaline would immediately make me feel confident and at home. Now I was terrified the entire time. My hands turned to stone, I couldn't catch a pass, couldn't shoot and felt like a fish out of water.

However, I did have one good game when we went to Kelowna to play the Wings. Fueled by contempt and anger for being traded, I lit up like I had in Revelstoke. But the moment I achieved a goal, I stopped working at it and I stopped trying. I didn't know it yet but that became my whole M.O. in life; "Just do enough to get there." At school, I would study for final exams the night before and manage to get fifty percent which was just enough to pass the year. I was lazy and lacked self-esteem. If procrastination had a tune, it was my theme song. I did as little as I could to get by.

For the next game after Kelowna, they moved me to the first line with Cliff Ronning and Craig Berube. These names should sound familiar as they both went on to have successful careers in the NHL. Next to them I shrunk, diminished, and choked. I didn't feel like I belonged there. It was an early-season game and I screwed up royally. I was especially intimidated playing with these guys and subsequently stopped trying altogether. I was benched part way through the game and in the stands for the next. To pour salt in my wounds, the team went on a road trip out East and they left me back in New Westminster.

"Okay." I thought when I found out. "That's fine. They don't need me and I don't need them. I quit!"

They didn't even single me out, they left other guys behind too. But in my self-centered way, it was all about me. Instead of buckling down, working hard and practising with the other guys who stayed back, I just folded and quit.

But what if I had treated it as an opportunity to turn things around instead? What if I had just seen it as motivation to focus, work harder and get my confidence back? I wasn't cut from the team, they had just brought the best players at the time. I still had a chance to earn a spot. It was similar to being sent down to the minors when you're in the NHL. Imagine one of those guys saying, "Well, you don't want me in the NHL, I quit," instead of working hard to get back there. This time, I failed to see it as a chance to grow, and laid down flat and admitted defeat. I went back to my old team in the SJHL where it was easier and more comfortable, giving up on what could have been a flourishing career.

Once back in Saskatchewan I started fighting instead of hiding. It started with one lucky fight: I beat up the toughest guy on the best team and word spread quickly. After that, I had a reputation as a tough guy. It was my second year in the league, I was seventeen years old and the games were easier.

I scored goal after goal and with my new reputation I should have felt triumphant, but on the inside, I was scared as hell.

Coaches would tell me, "You have the talent and the skill to make it to the next level, but you're not mature enough." After going back to North Battleford and playing a good portion of another season there, I gave up on that also. The coach was an asshole which took all the joy out of it. I returned to Sherwood Park Alberta to play for the Crusaders where Al Hamilton, former NHL'er, was the coach. He was such an awesome guy and a fantastic coach, he made playing a real pleasure again. I still keep in touch with him to this day.

I was offered three college scholarship to schools in the United States as a result of playing for Hammy. One was in Flagstaff, Arizona, one in Anchorage, Alaska, and one was at USIU in San Diego. I had always been interested in acting and had heard that the program at USIU was excellent. However, they said that the drama program would conflict with the hockey schedule and that I would have to choose another major. I didn't want to do that, so I looked into the radio and television program at NAIT in Edmonton. That also wasn't going to work, and I didn't have the best track record as far as studying was concerned which didn't help matters. I had barely made it through high school.

The truth was, nothing interested me as much as hockey and none of the programs at University stood out to me. The fact that hockey scouts were enthusiastic and offering me scholarships was, once again, the part that excited me the most. It was flattering and it also gave me some sense of what to do next; I was at a loss for what my future held. What was I going to do when I finished hockey? I had to face the facts, a future in the NHL was no longer within reach, so I might as well try to get an education.

I knew that I didn't want to go to school to become a lawyer or doctor or whatever it was that most people did. My academic skills were sub-par and had no area of focus whatsoever. It wasn't that I wasn't smart enough, it was simply that I did not apply myself and was lazy. Having been scouted made me feel more than a little cocky.

That self-centeredness and feeling of invincibility cost me. One day as I left the house heading to the rink my mom asked me, "You're going to put a visor on, aren't you?" I said, "Yes, I'm going to put one on tomorrow," and I meant it. The next thing I knew, I was in the warmup and we were doing 'three on two's — This is a drill when three forwards enter the offensive zone against two defensemen. Our centreman had the puck on the left wing, he passed it across for me to tap into the net, but our goalie shot his stick out to deflect it away. It was then that the puck went off his stick straight up into my left eye. I fell to the ice, put my hand up to my face as blood squirted through my fingers. Someone brought a towel and helped me skate to the dressing room. I tried to look at my eye in the mirror but Al Hamilton quickly sat me down and wouldn't let me look. A puck to the eye is what ended his NHL career. Someone ran off to call an ambulance and I was soon rushed off to the hospital.

On our way to the hospital, I blamed everyone apart from myself. I blamed God, I blamed the guy who passed the puck across, I blamed the goalie for deflecting it, but I should have blamed myself for not taking action when my mom told me to put the visor on. At the hospital, I had to have seventeen stitches above and below the eye. I was blind in that eye for well over a week and thought that I was going to lose sight in it permanently. I was angry and scared and thought the accident was going to be career-ending.

Miraculously, my eye healed and I was back on the ice one month later. I even continued, to some degree, to try to earn a college scholarship. This taught me a valuable lesson: don't tempt fate and be more safety-conscious. I could have lost sight in that eye, and even though I was angry about the incident initially, I was spared the loss of my eye. Now, I make sure I do the little things that only take a few seconds, like making sure I put on safety goggles or steel-toe boots when using tools or moving heavy equipment or furniture. It's a "do it anyway" moment in a slightly different context.

> *Think you can put it off until tomorrow?* "Do it anyway!"

CHAPTER 3

MODELING

We're flying over the Atlantic, mid-morning, with nothing but the blue, glistening sea below. The white noise and the cabin's compressed air have lulled my colleagues to sleep, but I'm awake in my seat, struggling to get a wink. Sometimes it's hard to grasp that my looks have got me here, travelling all over the world while getting paid. It should be enough to make anyone the happiest person in the world. So why is my anxiety constantly pumping away in my stomach? I press the button above my head, it lights up and as soon a flight attendant arrives, I ask for a double rum and coke.

In the end, college didn't pan out and by the time I was close to twenty, I was dabbling in commercial acting and moonlighting in a nightclub in Edmonton named *Goose Loonies*. The Alberta Drug and Alcohol Abuse Commission (ADAAC) had a TV commercial audition, and I ended up getting the role. It was like a public service announcement geared towards the prevention of drug and alcohol abuse. The irony was that I drank a lot, much more than I should. My buddy asked me, "Do they have any idea how much you drink?" I laughed and said, "Of course not!" One night at the club, a man in a suit approached me. He said that his name was Brian and that he was a scout from John Casablanca's modeling agency.

"Have you ever thought about giving modeling a try?" he asked me. I just chuckled and shook my head at first. But the more I thought about it, the more it sounded like a cool way to travel for a while and meet girls — something to do short term.

However, much to my surprise, I ended up spending about ten years in the field.

I began in Edmonton and Toronto. Then Japan and many parts of Europe, several additional Asian countries, South Africa, the US and Australia. It really was a wonderful way to see the world. When you have low self-esteem, you keep telling yourself that the next good thing that happens to you will finally make you happy. "If only I can get on that team, it will show everyone how capable I am."

"If I can have a hot girlfriend it will show everyone how desirable I am," and so on. There I was, young, tall, athletic and paid for the way I look. And yet I was still painfully shy and insecure. Whenever a big job came up, I would choke under the pressure of having to meet the people in charge, and the jeers of high school bullies would echo in my head, telling me I'm not worthy.

Despite getting a fair amount of work and remaining in the industry for a decade, my pattern of 'meeting the minimum requirements' was still in play. When I found myself in need of money I would go out and get some work. Then I'd have some money in the bank, and I would go off to somewhere like Thailand to sit on the beach and scuba dive for months on end. I would do that until I was broke again and would have to go back to work.

It was an immature way of thinking and certainly not the best way to manage a personal business. Similarly to hockey, I could have become more successful and done much more with it if I had executed properly. All the while, I still had that persistent shyness and insecurity which was an increasing concern. I wasn't outgrowing it because I wasn't changing my attitude or behavior.

One season I had the pleasure of walking the runway in several fashion shows during the Tokyo collections. Claude Montana, Hermes, Issey Miyake, Comme des Garçons, and a few other Japanese and international designers. Prior to one of the shows, I spotted large tubs of alcohol backstage. While I had mostly only drank alcohol socially and for fun, I had never used it as a crutch before. I thought it might actually take the edge off before heading out in front of hundreds of spectators and worldwide media.

I consumed half a bottle of vodka before the first show in under five minutes without a second thought. Within minutes my shoulders relaxed and the tightness in my gut loosened. When it was time to hit the runway I got out there and showed the collections off with ease. It was a real aha-moment. My friend Mr. Vodka was a constant companion at the collections. Who suddenly guzzles half a bottle of vodka and immediately feels calm and comfortable enough to appear cool and normal? Most people, especially young people, would have been virtually incapacitated if they downed ten to fifteen ounces of alcohol that fast, but I was just relaxed and in control.

Drinking was such a handy, readily available coping mechanism. And this is how I coped with general anxiety and the accompanying nervousness for years to come. I used alcohol as a crutch to hide my feelings, to stuff them down, and to make myself feel better. In fact, whenever I tried going through a "dry patch" my friends encouraged me to drink. I remember one of them saying he would buy the drinks for the night because I was "way more fun when drunk."

Starting from my younger teen years onward, I was self-absorbed and self-centered. I have a great many regrets around that, especially with my brothers. It wasn't just that I was wrapped up in myself and did my own thing, but others noticed and occasionally took offence at my attitude. Over the years the self-centeredness and drinking became worse.

One time, I was in a nightclub with my buddies and a woman who was four or five years older than us was literally screaming at me about how self-centered I was. I simply didn't care, I just looked at her, and walked away. But self-centeredness is also part of the disease of alcoholism.

Modeling provided me with some wonderful times. I met fantastic people and learned a great deal but, I was always looking for the next thing. I wasn't present, I wasn't enjoying where I was in the moment. Like a vagabond on an endless journey, I was always looking for the next thing. For example: I was based in Hamburg one late summer in the early '90s and had the great fortune of booking a two-week job for a Swedish catalogue which was shooting in Rhodes, Greece. Upon returning to Germany, the October chill set in. Since I hated feeling uncomfortable in any sense, I decided on a whim to go to South Africa. There was a travel agency across the street. With a plane ticket booked to Cape Town a few hours later, it wasn't long until Germany was a thing of the past. I ended up staying in South Africa for close to a year.

Cape Town with its white sand beaches, mountains and mix of cultures was amazing. The climate and the nightlife were nothing short of incredible, but these were the final days of apartheid. Tensions were high and the political situation made it too uncomfortable for me to live in.

My M.O. always dictated to do whatever was fun, whatever was irresponsible, whatever I could do to keep myself preoccupied and uncommitted. I was consistently chasing the next thing. In reality, all I was doing was chasing my own tail. And like a dog going 'round in circles, I could never catch it.

> *Don't want to choose the hard way over the easy?*
> "Do it anyway!"

CHAPTER 4

CAR SALES

As I look at myself in the men's room mirror, I splash water on my face to clear my head. The $400 bar tab is telling me it's time to go home. I can feel the keys to my brand new Lexus in my pocket. Another day, out drinking with the boys. It's been a long day and it's time to go home and face the music. Drunk again and I can't remember the last time I felt good.

I had worked as a model for nearly ten years and it was starting to bore me. Flying around the world didn't give me a buzz anymore and I was sick of living out of a suitcase. I wanted to move on and chase thrills somewhere else. I went home to Edmonton to visit friends. Shortly thereafter, a couple of us went out for a Tuesday evening drink and game of pool at the university pub. I ended up meeting a young lady. It was the woman who would become my wife and the mother of our three children.

Like the beginning of most new relationships, my time with her was like getting caught up in a whirlwind. We spent every waking hour together from when we met, sharing secrets and making promises we weren't going to keep. It was typical for me to act on a whim or run to or from something, always making split-second decisions. We had only been together for about three months when we went on holiday to Victoria, British Columbia. It was around Christmas and agreeably pleasant and mild on the island. We returned to a frigid -20°F Edmonton and instantly decided to move to Victoria.

I didn't have a job when I arrived there; I hadn't really planned that far ahead but, my father suggested that I should try my hand at selling cars. Coincidentally, my vehicle had broken down during the move, so that in itself was enough motivation to get into the car business. I applied to a couple of places and ended up at the local Toyota dealership. Sure enough, they gave me a car to drive. It solved both problems.

We were married within a year, had a son, then twin daughters a few years after that. I loved selling cars and found I had a knack for it. By all outward appearances, things looked great! I was on the sales floor for about four years until I was able to open a used car lot with a couple of business partners. After a few years the business went sideways because one of them was taking more than his share of the profits. By this point, I was a full-time smoker and my alcohol consumption had increased significantly. At that time, it wasn't much of an issue; I could drink, recover quickly and go to work without consequences.

It was a time when everything still looked great on paper. From an outsider's perspective, all aspects of my life seemed to be a huge success. I was making a lot of money but I still reverted to my usual M.O.; Not long after divorcing myself from the used car operation I was offered a job at a large Chevrolet dealership in Edmonton for a lot of money. So of course, I moved the family there. I worked there for nearly a year until one day, the general manager summoned me to his office moments after one of my friends had taken delivery of his new Corvette. The GM handed me a severance check, and fired me on the spot. They never told me the reason why but I am more than a little suspicious that it was due to my alcoholism. I was sober when hired and started drinking again a few months later. I hold no resentment whatsoever. On to the next store for a brief few months. It was then that the call came from an old boss and friend to fly to Calgary for an interview at the largest domestic retail store in Western Canada. Of course, my ego and the lure of the dollar were enough to uproot the family yet again and head south to Calgary. The interview consisted of getting drunk with the owner and the general sales manager. By that time, I was a professional drinker so of course, the interview went well. I really needed to stop drinking but how could I think of giving up something that seemed to work so well?

I would go between periods of excessive drinking and brief periods of sobriety. I sobered up again for a minute while we were living in Calgary, Alberta. My wife hated living there so I quit the job and we moved back to Edmonton. I took up the old job that I had previously left and I started drinking again. Over the course of a decade, I would be sober for two or three months, then drink for a year or two. Then I would be sober for six months, drink for a month. The last drinking stint lasted two and a half years. I was aware that the alcoholism was progressively getting worse but I lacked the commitment that it took to stop and stay sober. A couple of months after our return to Edmonton a sales manager position at one of the Toyota stores became available. This was home for the next six years. The longest stretch in a twenty-year career.

The entire time I was in the car business I had a multitude of different jobs, my resumé read more like a directory. I would leave half of them out if I was applying for a job or going for an interview. It would look like I was repeatedly getting fired or quitting. I would go whichever way the wind blew. Not that it wasn't true but I didn't want to appear that way.

Admittedly, it was a crazy way to live let alone raise a family. The allure was the jobs paid so much money that I would go from one high-paying job to the next. Working at the last Toyota store, I was making surgeon money. It was incredible how much they paid.

Looking at who I was on paper with the house, fancy cars, vacations, the clothes and whatever other luxuries I wanted, life appeared to be sensational on the outside. In reality, I was painfully unhappy, not to mention, terribly unhealthy, especially considering my age. On the inside, I was absolutely dying.

> *Not ready to look at your destructive behaviours?*
> "Do it anyway!"

CHAPTER 5

DIVINE INTERVENTION

The impact of my car hitting the ditch wakes me up from a drunken stupor. I'm still doing 60 mph as I crank the wheel to get myself back on the road. All day drinking at the lake and for some dumb reason I figured I could drive. The sheer fright of the situation gets me home on pure adrenaline.

In March of 2008 I took my family on a vacation to Mexico. At the time I had my hair bleached blonde with highlights. Vanity was alive and well. We were there for two weeks, and on the tenth day, my wife went on an excursion with a friend and I was left with the kids for the day. The girls were seven years old at the time and my son was nearly eleven. I applied sunscreen to them in the morning and let them play in the pool while I kicked back and had a drink. The hours went by and I kept ordering drinks with no intentions to stop. I was still watching my kids through the sunglasses, lulled by the alcohol into a false sense of security, telling myself they were perfectly safe. And then my twin girls got out of the pool, wanting a snack. "Daddy, my back stings," my daughter said. When I took my glasses off I saw that their skin was burnt to a crisp. I had forgotten to reapply sunscreen. My daughter flinched when I touched her skin, and I wanted to cry. "I'm so sorry," I whispered. I had to do a lot of apologizing later that day.

I rushed them up to the hotel room to get them out of the sun. I was already feeling ashamed about neglecting the kids when I saw my reflection in the bathroom mirror, drunk for the third time that day. I would drink, sober up, drink, and sober up. I just stared in the mirror at this bleach-blonde, bloated, glassy-red-eyed person. I had no idea who that guy was. Who had I become? Something inside of me changed, and at that moment I made one of the biggest decisions of my life. It was time to cut the booze once and for all.

It was a culmination of everything up to that point. It was the final straw; I was face-to-face with reality. While I was applying aloe vera gel to my kids' sunburnt skin, then suddenly seeing myself in the mirror — it made my skin crawl.

Of course, it was easier said than done. I ended up continuing to drink for the last few days of the trip. But this time it was different. We went back to Edmonton and I officially quit drinking for the final time. March 21, 2008 was the last day that I had a drink or drug of any type. By no means cured, but sober one day at a time and free of the compulsion to drink. I finally wanted to stop drinking more than I wanted to drink. The consequences of drinking had become increasingly worse. Alcoholism is a progressive illness, so every time I started drinking again, it didn't just pick up where I left off; it would be as if I had never stopped. I needed to make the decision that I wasn't going to stop for a month or two, and I had to crush the illusion that I could ever drink safely again. Once I finally smashed that notion, I could do the work that it took to become sober. I owe this all to my higher power who I choose to call God.

That was likely the most crucial turning point in my life, although I didn't have the desire or the skills to become physically healthy yet. I still smoked for another year, but I overcame that too. I read a book that helped me tremendously, *The Easy Way to Stop Smoking*, by Allen Carr. He was an old Englishman who has since passed away but reading his book and applying its message has kept me smoke-free to this day.

Over the years there have been countless times when I could attribute Divine Intervention to the only likely reason why I am still here. Despite that, it took many instances to come to the realization that I needed to stop and change something, on a very deep level. If I think about all the occasions when I drove drunk and had near misses in traffic or fell asleep at the wheel drunk, and woke up halfway into the ditch and pulled myself up back on to the road — it horrifies me. I'm thankful that nobody was hurt.

Back when I lived in South Africa in the early '90s, it was New Year's Eve, and my buddy and I were drinking all night. When it was time to head home from the party I volunteered to drive. My girlfriend at the time was in her car while I was driving my friend's car behind her. We went through an area where the locals were called Cape Coloureds. South Africans identified people as White, Africans, Indians, and Coloureds at that time. They're basically mixed-race people in this district, lighter skin Africans.

As we came around a corner, we encountered thousands of Cape Coloured people on the road celebrating. The area was packed. The light was just turning red, and my girlfriend ahead of us didn't stop at the light. She just drove right through. As a Canadian, I saw the red light and obediently stopped. Suddenly, all these young people, teenagers mostly, flooded towards us. Naively, I rolled my window down, "Hey, happy New Year." I said, but my buddy, Ernest exclaimed, "Grab the keys!" I was so confused. "What?" I said. "Grab the keys!" Ernest sternly insisted.

He reached across from his side and grabbed the keys as these people began to open the door. One guy pulled my seatbelt tight so I couldn't move. Another was trying to rip my watch off, and then I heard an agitated young man yell, "Who's got the knife? Who's got a gun?" Having no experience with this I just yelled out, "Whoa, whoa, whoa! Hey, hey, guys, I'm from Canada, we're just here visiting!"

I was half-panicking and half in disbelief. Next a young guy opened the rear door and tried to get in the back. Ernest reached back, roughly grabbed his arm and broke it! Then the adults that had seen what was going on came over, and a full-blown brawl ensued. People were fighting everywhere, now distracted with each other, Ernest gave me back the keys and it was our chance to get away. I put the keys in the ignition as fast as I could, and as bodies were literally bouncing off of the car I shot through the light to get out of there.

I felt that was divine intervention. They could have killed us because I hadn't been paying attention, was drunk, and had no business being there, but we managed to escape unharmed. It was a profound experience but I hadn't changed my behavior yet. I met a Christian lady while in South Africa, who asked me about my faith and I said, "You know, I had more faith growing up but it's waned somewhat." She said, "Oh, you're just on a walkabout," meaning I was finding my own way for a bit. She was right.

It reminded me of my mother who knew my lifestyle wasn't that of a good Christian. One of the things that she always used to say to me was, "God will never leave you. He'll be there, waiting for you." She was right.

There were so many times when the drinking was completely out of hand, when I fell down or got behind the wheel of a car. Often waking up wondering "Where am I?"

I remember one time when my son was ten, he said, "Dad, you look kind of green." I looked in the mirror and he wasn't kidding — my skin had a tinge of yellow/green. I'm sure that I had come close to the onset of cirrhosis of the liver or I was having liver failure. Luckily, I quit shortly after that.

There was a time in my youth when I was at a night club on a Monday night. The drink special was "three for one". I was supposed to meet my friends at another club on the opposite end of Edmonton so in preparation to head out, I had three or four triples before getting into my brother Mark's little yellow Plymouth Arrow.

The city had just made some road improvements and had changed the traffic lights in the West End as well as added a few new roads. I was looking at the light far in the distance and completely missed the one right in front of me. I ran the red light and rammed straight into the side of a car full of young people. The crash completely demolished my brother's car but thankfully, the passengers of the other vehicle were left unscathed.

The cop who arrived on the scene was my dad's cousin. By then, I was sitting in the back seat, surely reeking of alcohol. The adrenaline was pumping, so I wasn't slurring, when they asked me, "Have you had anything to drink?" and I boldly said, "No." They took me back to the police station. I waited an hour or two to call my dad to come and get me, which he did. Still to this day, I have never asked my dad what happened, but there were no consequences to my actions.

When Mark saw his totalled car, he said, "Man, you're lucky...." I knew I was; all I had was a scratch on my ankle. There were many indications that I should have quit drinking back then, but I kept getting through these incidents unharmed. At the time I could quit whenever I wanted to, but it was only temporary. My extreme vanity would kick in if I started to look like crap when I drank, so I could go days, weeks, or months without drinking if I needed to. However, in the end, it owned me and the choice to stop was removed.

There were many times when I managed to get away with things one way or another, or I would resort to dropping my dad's name, emphasizing he was RCMP. I was drinking amounts that frequently obliterated the legal limit as I had a very high tolerance right from the start. As much as Divine Intervention saved me, I think those situations enabled me to drink longer because there were no consequences. If the consequences would have been big enough, maybe I would've stopped sooner. But probably not.

> *Not willing to ask for help?* "Do it anyway!"

CHAPTER 6

TURNING POINT

Once your faith is restored, anything can be a church. A gym, a supermarket, nature.... I'm in Rome, Italy gorging on yet another pizza followed by gelato. I get back to the hotel and see a book on nutrition abandoned in the lobby. Back in the room I start to burn through the pages. My belly hangs over my belt and I realize I've got the textbook description of a dadbod. "I need to change my diet." It would have been a day without irregularities or quirks worth remembering. But the person who left the book in reception changed my life. When I put the book down, I was a different man. Maybe God was in the room.

There was another major turning point when I was in Italy in the year 2015 with my girlfriend at the time. She had to change her diet due to allergies, but I was still relatively unhealthy. I came across a book called *The Paleo Solution* by Robb Wolf in the lobby of our hotel. After reading it back in the room I decided to change my diet immediately. Within three or four days of cutting out all the garbage, the gluten and the processed foods, it significantly changed how I felt. Food is much cleaner in Europe than it is in North America. It also lacks the processing that most of our diet consists of. I mainly cut out bread and dairy, but I would still have gelato periodically — gelato is an absolute necessity when you're in Italy! There I was, in my late forties, and I simply decided to change; there was no lightning bolt epiphany. No "You're going to get a chronic disease if you don't change." It was more the case of, "All right, it's time to get fit again." I was fit in my twenties because I had to be to make a living. The twenty years in the car business were not conducive to living a healthy lifestyle. I smoked, drank, ate crappy food and worked in an ultra-high-stress industry. All by choice of course.

I started to feel better from the diet shift and that's when I began venturing into the tiny gym in our hotel. They had next to nothing in there; just a couple of dumbbells and a bench. I would work my way around the gym performing simple exercises then throw my running shoes on and run around the streets of Rome. That was how it started and I began to feel increasingly better. My girlfriend was the one who first told me about SEALFIT Kokoro, an intense military training camp that was designed to challenge civilians. She mentioned a man that she knew who was older than me and had completed the camp. This got me thinking, "If he could do it, why can't I?" I looked into SEALFIT training and read as much as I could, including retired Navy SEAL commander Mark Divine's book, *The Way of the SEAL*. Coach Divine is the founder of SEALFIT. The lessons learned reading his book made me realize that my attitude towards the military had been all wrong.

My mindset started to change as I read about the leadership skills that they develop in the military. I thought, "You know what? I didn't go to university; all I have is a high school diploma and a lot of what I learned was wrong. Most of what I know I learned while traveling. How was I going to learn the right way to live? How do you get through things when they're really hard? You just don't quit. You keep going.

This was a great contrast to my old mindset which was, "Oh, this is hard — I quit." There was always an excuse but now I wanted to lead by example.

Thinking back, I had wasted decades on decadence and I wanted to start over. There were some very difficult times. Such as the death of my brother and the breakdown of my marriage. My beloved little brother Mark passed away from colon cancer at the age of thirty-three. He was an incredible human being; loving, kind and gentle. He left behind his wife and three children. Needless to say my parents were devastated. At the time I dealt with the grief the same way I dealt with all emotional pain; I sought answers at the bottom of a bottle. No more excuses, onward.

After turning everything in my life around for the better, becoming healthier mentally, and physically stronger, I decided to push myself to another level. I decided to prepare for my first Kokoro camp. Kokoro 44 which was scheduled for the middle of July 2016. These events are held in the scorching heat in the high desert of sunny California. I had just turned forty-nine at this point and didn't know how to train for an event of this magnitude. I knew very little of Crossfit but had heard it was a great way to become strong and fit. I sourced the closest box and headed down for a Saturday morning intro class at Crossfit Viccity, in Victoria, British Columbia where I currently live. Cam Birtwell (owner of CFVC) hosted the class. I announced to him that I was going to attend Kokoro. He smirked at me and said, "Hey that's a great goal."

A couple of months later I mentioned it again and he repeated what he said the first time. In August of 2015, I approached Cam after a class and told him that I had signed up for Kokoro and asked if he would coach me. I guess that he finally believed me because he agreed to coach me twice a week. This soon became four times a week and shortly thereafter Cam joined in the workouts. We were training partners the entire year leading up to the event. I added solo running and rucking sessions to the schedule. I could not have completed Kokoro had it not been for Cam's knowledge and commitment to helping me. We remain good friends. I have the utmost respect for him.

July of 2016 neared. My good buddy Gary Haddon lives in Huntington Beach, California, so I planned to go down there early to hang out with him and his family. That way I could get acclimatized to the weather, drive to Temecula a day ahead, settle into the hotel, organize and prepare for the event.

Kokoro is touted as the "most powerful and challenging physical, mental and emotional training available to civilians in the world". They have based it on the regime used by the US Navy SEALs known as "Hell Week." Additionally, it combines the "Unbeatable Mind training" and "SEALFIT" program created by Mark Divine. It claims to be "the premier training event for forging mental toughness, emotional resiliency and elite team skills" according to their promotional material, which I can certainly attest to.

As luck would have it, on the flight from Canada to Orange County, I caught a chest cold. My nose was running like mad and I was coughing up mucus but I told myself: "Okay, no big deal. You still have a week before the event." However, the cold dragged on and wouldn't clear up. I started Kokoro at probably about sixty-five percent of my optimal health. I still had a lingering cough with wheezing in my chest, but I certainly wasn't about to start an event based on mental toughness by telling these Navy SEALs that, "Hey, I've got a bit of a cold." I simply powered through it.

In the end, I can't say how much the chest cold actually affected my performance. I'm sure it hindered me to some degree but, in subsequent events, I saw people sneezing and coughing and they pushed through too.

The evening before the event I was walking up and down the corridors of my hotel, thinking "What the hell was I thinking when I signed up?"

Kokoro is fifty hours of non-stop excruciating training with zero sleep. I had watched several videos, read all the after-action reports I could find, all the stories of people that have gone through this before, and I started to think, "Oh, what have I gotten myself into? I'm crazy. I'm an old man. I don't belong here with all these young guys. I'm going to get my ass handed to me!"

> *Do you think you are too old to change your life for the better?* "Do it anyway!"

Stair repeats
130 stairs steep incline
Choose 1 of the following
1. 20 rounds for time – 35 min cap

PART TWO

2. 15 rounds for time
w/ 22lb vest
15 push-ups at top
and bottom of stairs

3. Ruck on
carry 52lb sandbag
every second round

4. No ruck
- Farmer carry 2 53lb
kb for round 1.
- 2 71lb KB round 2
- weightless round 3
As many rounds as
possible in 50 mins

CHAPTER 7

KOKORO 44, FIRST 24 HOURS

It was the evening before Kokoro 44 and my nerves would not settle. "I'm a fifty-year-old recovering alcoholic, how am I going to complete an event of this magnitude?" I thought. "I'm in way over my head." Then I had an idea. I got in my rental car and drove thirty minutes to the event's location. It was near Temecula out in the high desert at Vail Lake. Having seen the videos, I knew the layout of the property. Out on the grinder (the concrete area where we did callisthenics) I did a few pull-ups at the rig that was set up then went down to the lake, walked around and got a feel for it. Getting myself situated calmed my nerves. I even sensed the tingling sensation of excitement in my stomach. Game on.

Back at my hotel, I had some food, and went to bed. The next morning, I opted for a taxi back out to Vail Lake so I wouldn't have to drive a vehicle to my hotel afterwards. The slippery leather of the back seat stuck to my legs as the Southern California heat was palpable.

I arrived slightly ahead of the scheduled 10:00 am check-in. Among the participants were a small busload of seven guys that regularly trained together.

We sized each other up while we introduced ourselves. They were buddies who knew each other well, and I felt like a bit of an outsider. (This was all in my head as usual.) I told myself I was going to do my best to work with them, despite being the outcast. We all signed in, gave our instructors our drivers' licenses, listed any medical issues and relevant information they requested. Safety was paramount; as true professionals the SEALFIT coaches wanted us to get the most out of it without getting hurt.

After the administration portion, we got a rundown of what to expect and things to watch out for. Rattlesnakes were one of them. That was enough to make my stomach turn. I have very few phobias, but snakes terrify me. I hate those things.

We could have roasted marshmallows in the sun it was so hot! Waiting to be told to drink would have been a death wish, so hydrating frequently was a top priority. We were given two canteens; one containing water and electrolytes and one with water only. I put one in each of the outer pockets of my Battle Dress Uniform pants (BDU's).

The first step in the event is the PST (physical standard tests): Which consisted of; a minimum of ten strict, AKA dead hang pull-ups, fifty push-ups, fifty sit-ups, fifty air squats, each in two-minute sets, and then run a mile in under nine and a half minutes in BDU's and boots. Another standard that must be met is completing a workout called "Murph." If you can't meet or exceed them you're out. Believe it or not, some people showed up unprepared to meet the standards.

I trained my ass off for hours on end to make sure I was over-prepared; I had a gruelling schedule of three days on, one day off, for almost a year. The off days would include hot yoga or a light run — something just to keep the blood flowing and increasing my mobility. On the training days, I would do CrossFit classes and frequent hikes up hills where I lived with a thirty-pound backpack on. Log PT, sandbag

PT, and thousands of push-ups. Hill sprints were a weekly staple while adding twenty push-ups and twenty squats at the base and top of the hill. Usual training sessions would last one to three hours. A typical training week consisted of ten to fifteen hours of strength, endurance, stamina, HIIT, and cold water exposure.

I would do the PT test *after* training so that I could hit the standards when I was fatigued. Many people would miss the standards because before you even get to them, you're beaten up for a couple of hours overheating in the sun with your nerves shot — that's exactly when you need to be able to hit them out of the park.

We had completed the first part of the PST test when the cadre sent us down to the shoreline. They told us to crawl through the mud and into the lake. I remember looking around and realizing that there was no hose, the only access to water was the lake. Fortunately, we would frequently use it to cool off.

Later in the afternoon we continued with the standards doing a workout called Murph, named after Lieutenant Michael Murphy, a Navy SEAL killed in Afghanistan. There's a book and movie about his story, called *Lone Survivor* starring Mark Wahlberg.

For the Murph workout, or "Body Armor" as Murphy called it, we were required to do 100 pull-ups, 200 push-ups, 300 squats, and a one-mile run on both ends of them while wearing a twenty-pound vest or a twenty-pound backpack. The maximum time allotted to complete it was seventy minutes. At the last minute they told us, "Because of the heat, you can do this 'slick,' meaning without the vest, but you've only got sixty minutes to complete it." We were assigned a partner and told to double the number of reps. Davis, my "swim buddy," was an incredibly fit young man who was training to become a Navy SEAL.

We had to work as a team, and only when both Davis and I completed each round were we able to move on to our next round of push-ups, pull-ups, and squats. As part of the standard requirement, you could only miss one standard. My mulligan was used up early. I had missed the pull-up standard by one. Somehow, I couldn't get my chin over the bar for the final rep. I just couldn't get the last one. Two strikes and you're out. Thankfully, I only had the one miss.

When it came time to complete Murph, I told Davis, "If we don't do this in under sixty minutes I'm going home." He understood my predicament, "Yeah, no problem. Piece of cake. We can do it."

The first one-mile run was a breeze and we were on track for a good score. We were competing with the other teams and I thought that we had a shot at winning the event. Next came the pull-ups, push-ups and squats. Davis kept missing the standard; he was not going all the way down or all the way up, and the cadres kept calling, "No rep. No rep." I had completed all my reps and was just waiting for him. He was built like a machine, but his form was all over the place.

When we finally got to the second one-mile run we had just under ten minutes to complete it. For some unfortunate reason my partner chose to not wear a hat. Most of us wore boonie hats which protected us from the direct sun. Avoiding overheating is critical. We started out running up a slight hill to the van, our halfway point. Just to be sure, one of the cadre was there to ensure that we ran the full distance.

About 300 yards into the run, Davis started walking, and I said, "Dude, come on, we got to go." But he was still walking! I yelled for him to start running and he managed a light jog. When we got to the turnaround point, he didn't look so good. We still had half a mile left to go and I was getting nervous.

Suddenly Davis took off ahead of me, moving swiftly. I thought, "Oh, perfect! He's got his second wind." I chased him down but then he veered off to the left toward the lake, but we needed to go right. I yelled, "Davis, this way!" Luckily, he heard me and we ran to where the cadre waited, stopwatch in hand. I chased closely behind him, but as soon as he crossed the line, he passed out.

Concerned, the cadre picked him up and dunked him in an ice bath to revive him. As he came to, he looked around and said, "Where am I? What day is it?" It was after talking to him for about 10 minutes that we were told we had made it under the time cap. But just barely before the cut-off.

I started tearing up thinking, "Oh my God, I made it through this!" Then it hit me, I'd made the standards, but now there were forty-plus hours to go. For a moment, the old me wanted to quit. Quickly I reminded myself of my WHY and the thought passed.

Davis, now revived, got back into the mix. Immediately more physical training began with some bear crawling and push-ups. Davis was not all there, mentally. The cadre were monitoring everyone closely and it didn't take long for them to make the call to med drop him. Just like that, Davis was out of the event.

Davis wasn't alone, everyone who couldn't meet the standards were dropped at that time. The cadre had allowed the guys that hadn't passed the standards to participate until approximately five or six o'clock in the evening. So at least they were able to experience six to eight hours of the fifty they'd signed up for.

The first night of suffering began at the beach in Encinitas. Rucking, running, playing leapfrog, bear crawling in and out of the water and laying prone in the surf. "Surf torture" is when you lay on your back, linking arms together while the waves pound over you. You can't see them coming. But as the cadre will tell you, over time you become "comfortable being uncomfortable."

I had done a lot of cold water training using the "Wim Hof method", so I was used to it, but many others were shivering involuntarily. I don't know how long that lasted exactly, but we were at it until the sun started to come up. At one point the cadre had us singing songs as the waves pounded over us. Myself and a fellow Canadian were told to sing our national anthem louder than our American teammates could sing theirs. We were significantly outnumbered but that didn't deter us. It was a lot of fun. After that it was back into the vans to head to Temecula once again, leaving Encinitas behind. My ears were ringing at this point and my eyelids felt heavier than ever before. We were not allowed to sleep for the entire fifty hours. Hell to pay if we did. Sleep deprivation was probably one of the hardest parts of the challenge.

The various training exercises, or "evolutions," were like mission simulations. During one of these evolutions, we were tasked to build a raft and swim across Vail Lake. We were given wood, ropes, and tires. Luckily Jim Steg, one of our teammates, was a home builder and we made the raft well under the time cap that we were given. While crossing the lake we had somebody in front dragging it, and took turns leading or pushing while holding on to the raft. The best swimmers, or those that weren't holding onto the raft, just swam. We were given the option to swim across the lake or to walk around it prior to the evolution. However, if you chose to walk, you had to carry everybody's gear. The guys who humped it were extremely tired by the time we arrived. Those of us that swam were refreshed by the one hour or so in the coolish lake. It was actually designed as a much needed break from the heat.

These evolutions are strategically mapped out by the cadre. Many were instructors at BUDS (Basic Underwater Demolition SEAL) located in Coronado, California. They know exactly how far to push, when to back off, and when to send us into the water to cool our core temperature. Safety always came first. Each evolution is extremely difficult mentally and physically but we knew the cadre were always on our side.

The lake evolution was followed by a "downed pilot" exercise, where we had to conduct a search-and-rescue operation for a lost pilot and carry him back on a stretcher. I really enjoyed the realism of that evolution and found it more exhilarating than challenging.

It was impossible to be aware of how much time passed. It was one evolution after the next. There was "Log PT" which consisted of a group of four or five people per log, following orders, such as overhead carry, left shoulder, right shoulder, squat, on your back, perform sit-ups with the log on your chest, lunge with it, and front-carry over a long distance. The logs weighed approximately 300 pounds, and we would have to carefully and efficiently carry the log and move as a unit. Log PT is designed to teach teamwork. It is manageable when everyone pulls their weight. Devastating if someone is sandbagging or shamming (dogging it). Everyone on the log knows it and so do the cadre, and they are not shy to single you out if you aren't carrying your share of the load.

Our boat crew consisted of a young fellow who is now a SEAL, an ex-collegiate swimmer from San Francisco, myself, and two others. We started with five, but partway through log PT, one guy suddenly quit. With one man down, that 300-pound log was heavier by twenty per cent. It might as well have weighed a million pounds as we held it over our heads and locked our arms out for stability until they told us otherwise. The sweat on our necks sizzled in the sun, the air vibrated. The intense focus, rhythmic breathing and persistent exertion had me entering an almost trance-like state. The log was the great equalizer.

These evolutions went on for hours. We were doing combinations of running, carrying sandbags, carrying each other, doing burpees, push-ups, bear crawls, and low crawls, all mapped out in a plan.

Next, they said, "Okay, now we want you to go fill up the sandbag until it's a third full," which was about thirty pounds, "and come back and put them in your backpacks. Here's your PVC weapon." It was a PVC pipe filled with sand, weighing ten to fifteen pounds. It was meant to simulate a rifle. "We're going on a hike." That night we went to Palomar Mountain, which was an eight-hour hike uphill with a thirty-pound pack on. It could have been gruelling all on its own, but as these evolutions keep going, it's the total combined exertion that begins to take its toll.

Later in the night, and before we went to Palomar Mountain, we started doing sprints, ran up and down hills, carried each other, buddy carries, as they call them, piggybacking and racing. In those moments, we were so focused on the tasks that we would lose track of time. Sometimes an evolution seemed to last for ten minutes, when in reality, some of them were two hours stints!

I don't know how long we had been going or what time it was, but sometime during the hike in the dark, sleep deprivation fully kicked in and the hallucinations started. Walking up a dirt road, the guy next to me said, "Hey, can you see the Teletubbies?" I said, "No but I see gargoyles on gold mansions." It was fascinating to witness how my mind was playing tricks on me; I'll never forget it. The weird thing was I knew I was hallucinating but that didn't stop them from happening.

Then one guy said, "Do you see that snake?" Another guy confirmed, "Yeah." Then I thought, "Uh-oh." The three of us had seen it. This was not a hallucination.

Its long, fat body, keeled scales, and triangular head didn't leave much to doubt: on the other side of the hill, a rattlesnake was observing us with its cat-like eyes.

As we turned to look at it, it bolted up the hill. Luckily, it was more afraid of us than we were of it.

> *Don't want to get off the couch? "Do it anyway!"*

INSIGHTS:

1. Show up early
2. Make a decision, then commit to it
3. Get acquainted with your fears and visualize conquering them
4. Push past your comfort zone and keep going
5. Train for success
6. Over-preparation builds confidence
7. Don't let the fear of something be greater than the reality of it
8. Tell yourself you will always do your best work, no matter the obstacles

9. Train harder than you will need to execute the task
10. Accept your flaws, then change them
11. In life you don't get endless shots, so each one has to count
12. When in doubt, drink water

CHAPTER 8.

KOKORO 44, SECOND NIGHT

As we caught a glimpse of the summit of Palomar Mountain, a very lean young fellow who was a distance runner in college and now a SEAL, collapsed on the ground with a groan. "Hey man, are you OK?" we asked while rushing to check his pulse. Luckily, one of the guys was a doctor and decided he was fine, just exhausted. It was time he admit defeat. We had to carry him, his pack and his weapon up the remainder of the hill. Unfortunately, we didn't make it on time. We had been given a mission that we were supposed to accomplish, but we failed. Yet we did the right thing by carrying our teammate and staying together.

The cadre sat him in the van once we got to the top and said to the rest of us, "All right. Put all your gear in the vehicle and run back down the hill." It was pitch black, there were holes everywhere, rocks strewn about, and guys started to fall as they ran. My knees were totally lit up so I didn't run very fast. My buddy Raul Rodriguez and I stuck together, (Raul and I keep in touch often. As mentioned, we made lifelong friends that weekend.) Fortunately, people only suffered minor injuries.

We ran downhill to a specific point where the coaches were waiting. Then out came the stretchers. Boat crews of seven were organized. In each crew, they would select the heaviest guy and say, "Okay, he's injured. Down he goes." The injured had to be loaded onto the stretcher and carried to the next checkpoint. Four of us carried him. One on each corner. After many failed attempts to carry the stretcher for more than a few seconds at a time we came up with a plan. One guy carried the weapons, four on the stretcher, and one person resting. Swapping out as needed. We were exhausted yet continued down the mountain for hours in the darkness. It was absolutely brutal.

At the next checkpoint the cadre said, "Okay, stretchers in the van, backpacks on, weapons in hand. You have twenty minutes to make it to the exfiltration point where a helicopter is waiting. Go!" We did a light jog to get to that point, but I have no idea how long it took.

Upon arrival the cadre screamed at us, "You went too slow, you missed it! Now you're going to have to go to checkpoint B. If you miss it, there's going to be hell to pay." Then they ordered us to drop into the lean and rest (extended arm plank) in a single file on the gravel road and put our feet on the person's shoulders behind us. That was the penalty, and we didn't want to do it twice. It was awkward, humiliating, and took us several tries to get it right.

We took off at what felt like a sprint. My heart was absolutely pounding out of my chest. I said a prayer asking God to protect it from bursting. It felt like we ran forever but running at that pace, it must have taken about half an hour to finally reach the van. At the van one of the cadre gave us directions starting with, "Stay there…" The rest of the directions were a blur but after standing there for a while, waiting for additional orders, we debated what to do next. The order could have meant "wait for further instructions" or "get in the vans when you arrive." We all just said, "Fuck it," and got in the back of the van. That was exactly what we were meant to do. They were waiting for us to make a decision as a team before driving us back to Temecula.

As we drove back, the sun was coming up; a glorious sign that it was all nearly over.

It must have been six or seven AM and we'd only have to make it until noon. Then a euphoric feeling kicked in; we had made it. Or had we?

Just when we thought we had found our last spurt of motivation to carry us to the end, knowing there were only five or six hours left, they told us, "We're probably going to go longer. You haven't earned this; you're not working as a team. We're going to carry on." After that they ramped up the intensity. We crawled, low crawled, and high crawled through the dirt and gravel. Then straight into an ice bath. Mark Divine arrived shortly thereafter.

Coach Divine had a nineteen-year career as an active duty and reserve Navy SEAL. We had no idea what to expect and were pleasantly surprised when we were each given a yoga mat. We did some light stretching and yoga while he went around to each one of us, asking about our experience during the event. What had we learned? In what ways had we grown? What would we take away from the experience?

It still wasn't over... Next up was what we believed to be the last evolution. We had to gather around a large pile of rocks while coach Divine shared different mental toughness techniques, and some of his experiences, in the hopes that we would apply the lessons to our regular life; we had pushed well past our perceived limits. I hadn't yet experienced what they refer to as a "Kokoro moment", which is the merging of the heart and mind.

As we awaited our next challenge, one of the head coaches named Lance Cummings called out, "Harlow..." he said it aloud, but not directly at me. "There you go, giving an 80% effort just like the rest of your life."

It was like a punch in the face and I thought, "Oh my God, he just called me out on my life long M.O.!" He was right. All I had ever done was put in as much effort as I needed to get by. In school. While playing hockey. Modeling. I had never dared to give one hundred percent. This guy, who didn't even know me, had called me out on my worst flaw.

To start the rock evolution, coach Divine said, "Choose a rock that describes you and your will. If you pick a rock that's too big, your ego's too big. If you pick one too small, you don't think enough of yourself." With that in mind, I looked at this heap of rocks, "Oh, there we go. The perfect rock." I picked it up. It weighed about forty pounds.

We had to carry the rock from the pile across a 300 yard field, up a long, steep hill, and around and down the other side back to where we started. Approximately three miles. It was easily 110 degrees by then. Meanwhile, one of our team mates had lost or forgotten his hat. Since we were supposed to be working as a team at this point, coach Cummings made us all remove our hats. So off came the hats. Teamwork always! Holy shit, was it hot!

I was one of the last to choose a rock. While I was carrying it, Mark Divine walked up behind me and said, "Harlow, why is your rock so small? Why is Steele's rock so much bigger?" I said, "I don't know. Maybe he thinks more of himself." Which of course was the wrong answer. Steele is an absolute stud and I was not taking a shot at him but I couldn't think of anything else to say. "Switch rocks!" he yelled at Steele and me. His was a slab! It was about three or four inches thick, and about two feet long by three feet. I could barely lift it off of the ground.

Eventually, I managed to hoist it onto my shoulder and take a few steps. It felt like the rock was driving me into the ground. I knew I wasn't allowed to put it down, so I'd bend over while holding it on my lap in order to steal a quick break. I was huffing and puffing like a freight train. "Get it up. Harlow, get that rock up!" commanded Mark Divine calmly and directly. He had no need to raise his voice. The man isn't named Cyborg for nothing.

I would raise the rock to my shoulder, take a step or two, then — boom! I'd tilt back down, lift it up once more, take a few more steps, then back down it'd go. I was trying to switch from shoulder to shoulder, but it was just too heavy. I thought, "I'm never going to make this. I'm going to fucking fail Kokoro in the final two hours over a stupid rock!"

Looking me square in the face, Coach Divine stopped and said, "I'm going to show you how to breathe. It's all about breath control. Okay, in through your nose, out through your mouth." I continued the exercise following his guidance until it calmed me down.

"Okay, now move." I continued to breathe as directed and hoisted the rock onto my shoulder effortlessly. As I started to walk, now in control of my breath, Coach Divine began reciting positive mantras for me to repeat. With each step he would say "You got this," "Piece of cake," "Hooyah." My negative thoughts were replaced with positive affirmations. "I got this." I had breath control; we walked up the hill and I was able to switch the rock from shoulder to shoulder with ease. At the top, I was in awe. The transformation from unbearably strenuous to total ease was absolutely incredible. You really can control the body and mind using breath control and positive mantras. This was a real eye-opener to me and a tremendous breakthrough!

As I started down the hill, one of our teammates was laying on the ground. I wasn't sure if he was injured or resting. He was lying beside his rock, surrounded by several coaches. They were barking at him "Get up! Get your ass off the ground!" No mercy. The sheer will and tenacity that this man demonstrated was awe inspiring. His rock was at least thirty pounds heavier than mine yet he picked himself up off the ground, battled with his huge chunk of stone and we slowly walked down the hill with our heads held high.

When we eventually caught up with the rest of the team that was waiting at the bottom of the hill, the cadre told the others what had happened and our rocks were immediately exchanged with more manageable ones. It was a lesson in teamwork and cooperation. It takes a village.

The brief time spent one on one with coach Divine was life-changing. He taught me how to calm my body and mind by practicing breath control and verbalizing positive mantras.

These techniques activate the parasympathetic nervous system which counteracts the sympathetic nervous system AKA the fight-or-flight response. This experience was the single most valuable takeaway of the entire event and helped unlock my inner strength. I use this technique daily, especially when training, and during ultra-endurance events. I have passed this knowledge on to many clients and friends as an applicable tool for coping with any stressful situation.

I thank Coach Divine for the biggest "Aha moment" of my first Kokoro event. I am forever grateful to him for that gift.

After the rock evolution, we formed two groups on the grinder for more log PT. Coach Divine faced us. The rest of the cadre flanked him. We were then asked, "Who knows the SEAL code?" Nobody answered. He asked again, "You mean to tell me none of you guys took the time to learn the SEAL code?" Fortunately, I had learned it after reading a prior participant's action report or AAR. It said that it was something you "may need to know." I am certain that the others would have had it memorized had they known. Truth be told, I memorized it out of fear of the consequences.

"Overhead carry, move!" coach Divine yelled.

Remembering there are seven points, I exclaimed loudly that I knew the code.

"Okay, what's the first one?"

"Loyalty to Country, Team and Teammate."

"Correct! What's the second?"

I searched my mind for it and called out: "Serve with Honor and Integrity On and Off the Battlefield."

My shoulders were burning as we kept the logs over our heads.

"Continue!" shouted Divine.

"Ready to Lead, Ready to Follow, Never Quit," I grunted.

"Take responsibility for your actions and the actions of your teammates."

As I called out each line, coach Divine explained the meaning behind the words.

"Excel..." I started, but my mind was foggy.

"Excel as Warriors..." Coach Divine helped.

"Excel as Warriors through Discipline and Innovation!"

"Train for War, Fight to Win, Defeat our Nation's Enemies."

We continued to maneuver the log as he explained the code: Overhead carry, squat, left shoulder, right shoulder! Over and over!

Finally, I exclaimed the seventh line:

"Earn your Trident every day."

The coach had everybody echoing his booming voice, "Hooyah!! Hooyah!! Hooyah!!" Finally, he exclaimed, "KOKORO 44, YOU ARE NOW SECURED!"

We let the logs hit the ground like a sack of bricks. I was crying, the other guys were crying. I should have been in so much pain. But then and there I couldn't feel the cuts on my hands or arms, my feet throbbing, the muscles aching or the hunger pangs. I hadn't slept for two days but I felt as if I was reborn. My body and mind were truly connected in a state of euphoria. The birth of my children aside, it was the most incredible feeling of my life, better than any sport or hockey game win that I had ever experienced. My life had changed, and I would never be the same. I was not my past; I was a new me.

> *Don't want to venture out of your comfort zone?*
> *"Do it anyway!"*

INSIGHTS:

1. Team work makes the dream work
2. Find the takeaway in all experiences
3. You're only as strong as the weakest link
4. Look after your team
5. Not everyone is going to make it
6. Surround yourself with people willing to push your limits
7. Find comfort in discomfort
8. When working in a team, the only way you win is when everyone wins
9. Find ways to have fun challenging yourself
10. Look for your own Kokoro moments in life
11. When the finish line is in sight, push harder
12. With breath control and positive affirmations, you can push your body and mind further than you thought possible

CHAPTER 9

KOKORO 51

Life after the first Kokoro became easier; I frequently thought about the accomplishment of completing Kokoro 44. I decided to become a coach to help others transform themselves. I took my level one CrossFit certification and learned as much as I could through reading and watching other coaches. I wanted to help people like me become fit — take their health and fitness back. I started K44FIT which was modeled after Kokoro 44. We developed the website and I started doing bootcamps on the beach and in parks, in and around Victoria, BC and built a following.

However, it was not yet the type of training that I wanted to do.

For the next phase of my coaching, I began coaching twelve-hour crucibles along the lines of SEALFIT. I wanted to encourage and train people to participate in Kokoro. Cam from CrossFit VicCity co-coached the first twelve-hour crucible. Seven people participated in the inaugural event.

A group of eleven businessmen from Edmonton came out for the second one. Then many of their wives and girlfriends flew out for a private twelve-hour crucible and they crushed it! It was during that year when I was also training my friend, Nathan, for Kokoro, that I realized I needed to sign-up again.

July, 2018 I participated in Kokoro 51. Once again it took place in Temecula and the Vail Lake area, only a slightly different spot. This location had a much more rugged terrain, with steeper hills and more of them.

Generally speaking, it was a similar format as the previous one. We all arrived for the sign-in and introduction. This time there were more people; twenty-six of us to be exact.

If you lined everyone up and asked me to pick the twelve people who would finish the event, I'm certain I would have been eighty percent wrong. Some of the fittest people attending, including one who was on the TV show *The*

Bachelor, became dehydrated, couldn't keep anything down, vomited everywhere and had to tap out on day one.

You would think that a retired professional MMA fighter, who I thought was incredibly fit, would make it through to the end. Nope. He cramped up on Palomar mountain and couldn't make it, also due to dehydration. There are many factors involved in surviving and completing Kokoro, but appearance isn't one of them.

A great deal of it is a person's strength, endurance and cardio fitness level. But the mental toughness is the most critical component, as is the gear preparation. In addition to that, there's nutrition and hydration, which is something you have a lot of control over.

When we arrived, it was excessively hot. I love the heat. In that regard, nothing had changed since Kokoro 44. We stood in the shade while we could, and having been there before, I obviously knew what to expect. I felt confident and calm. I was already having fun; laughing and joking but you could see the fear on everyone's faces. After a year of training with my buddy Nathan, I was confident that we were prepared.

The cadre had us lined up for more than half an hour just waiting. This is designed to create fear as we over-think what awaits us. Nathan was as nervous as I was at Kokoro

44. The mind games start right from the beginning. One of the things we were supposed to do during check-in was to give them our gear, our backpack or whatever else we had. One guy was so nervous that he forgot and was standing in line with his backpack on until somebody asked, "Why do you have your pack on?" He looked around panic-stricken and blurted out, "Uh-oh, I'm fucked; I'm so fucked." Then of course the first thing the cadre do is zero in on him. He's got his backpack on, not paying attention to detail, and so he's not going to live that down. "We're going to call you 'Backpack' from here on in".

The cadre had him crawl into the ice bath and roll around in the mud with his backpack on. It didn't take him long to quit. Those are the types of things that they will do to hone in on you if you want to be different or you don't want to be part of the team. They'll single you out and make you suffer.

To kick things off and get us warmed up, we ran a circuit in the hills. We did low crawls through the dirt and the gravel, crawling on our bellies wearing long pants with only t-shirts on top. With chafed arms and sand lodged down our pants we stood up and ran back to the starting point.

Once back at the start it was time for the welcome party. We stood in formation in rows of five, a few feet apart. Next, the hoses came out to cool us down. After we had a quick rinse we went straight into burpees, push-ups, sit-ups, leg levers, bear crawls, and low crawls for hours in the heat and mud. I had learned to absolutely love the intensity. There was also the added satisfaction of being able to meet the physical and mental challenges with a smile and not be out of breath — this time around it was fun. We had trained extremely hard and I was in much better shape than at Kokoro 44. The countless hours of training had paid off!

After the "fun" start, we had to complete the standards just like Kokoro 44. It's the minimum set of requirements, so it's something that has to happen at each event. Again, some people just couldn't make it. Especially after several hours of PT. You absolutely must be able to meet the standards when fatigued. You are fooling yourself if you think training at home or in an airconditioned gym with the music playing will prepare you for an event like this.

With the PST finished, we went for another run. We ran along a winding gravel path with a steep hill off to one side. One of the primary purposes of these events is to teach teamwork and leadership. Individuals don't last. You soon learn that on our own, we don't do as well as when we pool our efforts.

Some have made it through being 'lone rangers,' but the difference between surviving the event and excelling is apparent. When I did Kokoro 44, I just wanted to survive and complete it. At Kokoro 51, I wanted to become a better team player, a better leader, and help as many people get through it as I could. That was a big part of my WHY.

For the next evolution we had to run up and down a long, steep hill as a team. They asked us how long we thought it would take us as a group to run up to the top, turn around, and come back down. We guessed a time and they said, "Okay, we'll start there." Once we got back, they would give us a time-hack. If we hadn't met it, we'd have to do it again — as many times as it took. As we repeated the exercise trying to get it right, people were passing out, falling over, and dropping off in great part due to the heat. It was still well over 100 degrees.

At one point in the evolution one of the coaches turned to me and asked, "Harlow, how old are you?" I said, "Fifty-two," then he called to one of the other guys, "How old are you?" The guy replied, "Twenty-two". The coach looked back at me and said, "Good for you; age is just a number." I said, "I love this shit, Coach," he started laughing and made us run up the hill again!

Looking back at my life it blows my mind that today I absolutely thrive in these situations. I just love to push myself past my perceived limits because once I do, those limits get stretched even further and I'm capable of doing more. It's an addiction that I welcome and much healthier than the old ones. If you can call it an addiction? No matter... Kokoro 44 really turned my life around as far as pushing the bar farther than I ever thought it could be. Things were still daunting, but I knew they were manageable. I was prepared for the pain and discomfort. I knew it would suck but I also knew I would get through it like I had before.

The first evolutions were much the same as Kokoro 44. Some parts were a little different but generally speaking it was similar. One of the new evolutions was the cargo van pull. The cadre attached a tow rope and made us pull the van for hours. The driver would apply the brakes to make things a little more challenging whenever it suited him. Probably more for his amusement than anything. We lugged the van through a campground filled with curious onlookers and across a field next to a swimming pool. Once the cadre decided that we had played human tow trucks for long enough we had a quick water break. We were separated into four-man boat crews for the next evolution. We had team events where we had to carry each other while running and bear crawling with a teammate on our backs.

"It pays to be a winner." A phrase said many times by the cadre. It means win or pay the price. Our boat crews were selected by height. Our boat crew consisted of a young fellow, now a Canadian Special Forces soldier, two young German guys, and myself. We kept winning every event, whether we had to carry each other, run, or bear crawl. It didn't matter. We had decided to win and nothing was going to stop us. We were all extremely competitive on our team. Every time we'd win, we were able to sit back and rest, as of course… it pays to be a winner. The other guys would have to keep working, and my buddy Nathan later told me that it was his darkest hour and he seriously considered quitting.

Once we completed the team events, we went to the pool and swam which was refreshing and reinvigorating. When we went to the pool during the first Kokoro, I found it tough, but going into Kokoro 51, at approximately ten pounds lighter and leaner, I was able to run and swim more efficiently. The training had made me better at everything across the board.

After the afternoon's "evolutions," it came time to do Murph. We lost a few more people during Murph. This time we wore twenty- to thirty-pound packs and were allowed 70 minutes to complete the workout. The guy from *The Bachelor* began vomiting and couldn't keep anything down. Dehydration was starting to set in for many and our numbers dwindled rapidly. The intensity level was much higher on day one than at Kokoro 44. I believe that it may be because we had access to water more readily and the danger of heatstroke was minimized. It was also possibly done in order to weed people out sooner and whittle it down to the number most likely to finish. The prepared made it through. Attention to detail is also paramount. When the cadre gave us orders to drink some of us downed as much as we could, others sipped. The people that didn't do as directed went home as dehydration takes out more participants than anything else. After Murph, which was about eight or twelve hours in, we were given our first snack: a protein bar. This was also new to me. We ate as often as we wanted to at Kokoro 44. Luckily, Nathan and I had trained in a fasted state regularly.

Unlike Kokoro 44 where we went to the ocean the first night, then did the hike on the second, at Kokoro 51 we hiked on the first night. It made more sense this way, because the second night we were almost delirious, and it's almost futile to attempt to push us that hard afterward. We ascended Palomar at such a rapid pace that it took out more people than the heat and dehydration combined.

Quitters had to get in the "Loser Van," and sit and watch as everybody else continued. Then those continuing would get in the van and together we would all ride back. That heavy feeling of regret must have been incredibly burdensome for the quitters. I certainly felt for them.

When we hiked to the top of the hill it was getting close to daylight. We still had to run back down but this time we didn't have to carry anything or anybody. It was a very straight-forward jog all the way down. As the sun came up, it was an awe-inspiring moment; just beautiful. We could see the ocean from the top of Palomar Mountain; it was breathtaking. When we arrived at the vans the sun had fully risen. It was a quiet drive back to Temecula. Heads back, mouths open. I stayed awake anticipating a beatdown that never came. We must have had a more lenient cadre driving.

SEALFIT hosts events that are similar to Kokoro but shorter in duration. The 20X is twelve hours and the 20XL is twenty-four hours. These events were to run parallel to ours. So at what must have been almost 10pm on Saturday, night two for us, the participants for 20X and 20XL began to show up. What we didn't know was they had arranged giant spotlights that faced the grinder, a large dirt area. The spotlights shone directly on us as we assembled for our second welcome party. Then the hose came out, and it was time for another beat down! More push-ups, burpees, squats, low crawls, bear crawls, on your front, on your feet, and on your back! Into the ice bath, roll in the mud, move, move, move!

We repeated the exercises as instructed completely drenched and muddy. I can't speak for the others, but I was having a blast, a big smile on my face. What we didn't know was the cadre had the 20X and 20XL men and women sitting just beyond the spotlights, watching us.

When that finished, we all went and sat by the fire in a row which they descriptively call, "nuts to butts" if you can picture that. Mark Divine began to speak. We could see the terrified expressions on the faces of these new guys and gals after watching the shit-kicking we had just taken. They knew that they were up next. Mark Divine gave an inspiring speech about teamwork, leadership, and the importance of knowing your WHY. This only prolonged the inevitable, while we sat by the fire. The temperature had dropped and it became quite chilly.

Coach Divine had stopped by our group earlier as we had a rare break in the action. We were resting in the shade as he made a point of saying hello to each of us. He looked at me and said, "I recognize you." "Yeah, Kokoro 44," I told him. "Did you graduate?" he questioned. Yes was the answer. "And you're back?" he asked. Some of the other coaches had said the same thing, "What? You're back again? Are you crazy?" I told him about my first Kokoro experience and how I went as an individual just trying to get through, but this time I wanted to be a better team player.

We'd already been going for over thirty hours when the cadre told us that all three groups were going to run a race. To the 20X and 20XL participants they said, "If anyone from the Kokoro group beat you there's going to be hell to pay." Then the coaches came to us and said, "You better not let any of these 20xer's beat you." I didn't bust my ass to run super-fast, but I still finished ahead of many of them. I didn't feel the need to win. Old bull theory. A big group of our people beat their guys by a noticeable amount, even after thirty hours of arduous work! The 20xers received the pounding they were promised! Once that was finished, they were essentially inaugurated into the event.

Next, we piled into vans and drove just over an hour to the beach. There we were subjected to more hours of running, sandbag carrying, and something called 'sugar cookies.' To make a sugar cookie you run into the ocean, get nice and wet, then find a spot on the beach where the sand is the softest, and roll around until fully coated. No bare skin must be visible. The penalty was repeating the process until we got it right. It was down my back, in my pants, in my face, in my ears. I was picking sand out of places for weeks!

Surf torture was a different experience this time. I was shivering so much my teeth were chattering. It might have been because I was ten pounds lighter or possibly because the ocean was actually colder. Most likely because we did not train for it. I noticed it wasn't as bad when I was completely submerged in the ocean and was worse when we had to dive into it, get up and run back. The X'ers were all there as well now and we collectively took a pounding for another hour or two.

We linked arms and lay on the beach so that when the waves came up, they would only cover an inch of our bodies before retreating. I would start to tremble as the waves returned for another round of chilling. I was becoming colder by the minute. I remember looking up at the clouds as they appeared to be changing shape, in more ways than normal. I had begun to hallucinate.

We were then told to walk knee deep into the ocean, link arms, and take seats. The ocean seemed to become angrier as time moved on. The waves were stronger, undercurrents intensified and I was starting to question why I was putting myself through this shit. With the three groups together, there were probably about forty people linking arms. Every now and then one side of the chain would get dragged into the ocean while everyone held on as tightly as they could. Some were having more difficulty than others and had to scramble to get back to the chain of bodies when the link broke.

It was reassuring to know that two medics and a doctor were at the ready. When getting a med check, we were told to raise our arms above our heads and look straight ahead while they shone a light in our eyes. We were asked questions in order to determine our level of cognitive function. They were frequently testing for hypothermia. Every time we returned from the water, they would check us.

I kept arguing with myself, "That's it. Fuck it. If they put us in the water one more time, I'm going to quit." This is where the teamwork mentality during Kokoro really makes the difference between winning and losing. We went back into the water yet again and I had my arms linked with my teammates on either side. I said, "Look, I've done this before. I'm freezing my ass off. I think I'm going to tap out." They said, "No, you're not. This is going to end soon." They talked me out of it, thankfully. It was a great benefit having that support present to keep me in it and push through.

The power of teamwork is an incredible asset to help persevere and power through the most difficult challenges. That was the only time during Kokoro 51 that I really wanted to quit. I remember thinking to myself, "What do I have to prove?" Opening the quit door is a slippery slope. I was talking to myself, weighing the pros and cons, and it surprised me how I probably would have quit this time, had those guys not been there to encourage me. It is a humbling realization.

Once out of the water for the final time, we began our next evolution carrying sandbags while running up and down the steps between the condominiums above the beach. The coaches were adamant about us not talking. It had to be done in total silence so that we didn't disturb the neighbors. It was impressive to have a huge group of people like that running up and down carrying sandbags and racing. We had time limits to meet which must be completed in absolute silence — it was another example of discipline and teamwork.

Then as we got back to the beach, I thought I was hallucinating again. There was a 350-pound Hawaiian man dressed in drag riding down the beach on a bicycle. I wasn't certain if my eyes were deceiving me or not so I asked the other guys, having remembered my experience at the first Kokoro, "Hey, do you guys see the guy on the bike?" "Yeah," they said. Relieved, I replied, "Okay, good; I'm not hallucinating!" At 3 am, in the dark, he was quite the spectacle to see appearing seemingly out of nowhere!

When we were finished on the beach, the Kokoro participants hopped into the vans and went for breakfast. The 20xers went straight back to Temecula. We were fed a hearty meal in a freezing cold restaurant, while we were still soaking wet. We knew the end was in sight but the cadre were sure to remind us, "Look, you're not done, yet."

With full stomachs and after a short drive, we started running up and down hills again, this time in the heat of the sun. The temperature was back up to 110 degrees. It was actually hotter on Sunday than it had been on Friday or Saturday. While we were running, one guy had to bail because he fell and injured himself. Then one of the youngest lads collapsed. He had passed out due to heat exhaustion and they had to put him in an ice bath to revive him. He was a SEAL candidate and he knew we were close to the finish line. The cadre told him, "Okay, I'm sorry, man, for safety, we're going to have to med drop you." He jumped out of the ice bath and said, "Fuck that!" He had no shoes or boots on and just jumped into the final beatdown with us and said, "You're not taking me out of this!"

I remember this clearly and thought, "Good for him!" I have no idea if he actually became a SEAL or not. If he maintained the mindset that he displayed at Kokoro my money is on him. There was one other guy who was really waning towards the end who was also a SEAL candidate, and he hung in there also.

They continued our beat down with crazy PT in the mid day heat. The 20X and 20XL groups had joined us again. We were on the grinder doing burpees, yelling, screaming, doing push-ups, rolling, doing squats, all at a feverish pace and then BOOM! They secured us! It was over.

I immediately looked for my buddy Nathan to give him a hug, but he had run over to congratulate the 20xers. All he heard was that 20X was secure; he hadn't heard it was us as well. He thought it was still game on! I gave him a big hug and said, "We made it!" and he looked at me confused, "What do you mean? It's just the 20xers." I told him, "No, all of us!" Then the tears just started flowing, for both of us! It's hard not to get emotional after what you go through in an extreme event like these.

I was so happy for him. He had been through so much in the year leading up to the event and required a ton of physical therapy just be able to attend. It was awesome for the two of us to train together, and so gratifying to get through it. Nathan is one of the most mentally tough individuals that I know. He went into the event with old hardware in his knee which required surgery not long after the event.

Some of the others that completed the event include a young Irish woman who lives in Dubai, a strong young kid from New York with a great sense of humor, Sam the Aussie, the two SEAL candidates and a smattering of others. Despite outward appearances, this group had not just the physical capabilities, but the mental toughness to succeed and not quit when others did. It was a great feeling and highly rewarding to have several teammates come up and thank me for helping them get through to the end. My reason for attending Kokoro 51 was validated and I feel like a better human being because of it. It was a humbling experience.

I don't feel like this event held a specific "Kokoro moment" like at Kokoro 44 during the rock evolution, but a definite highlight was when the coach looked over at me and asked my age. I remember how much I was thoroughly enjoying myself and truly thriving in that moment. Age really is just a number.

As mentioned previously, I had trained harder this time around and went in more lean, which definitely helped meet the physical demands. Knowing what to expect was a bonus because I was able to prepare better mentally for what was in store. All of these aspects allowed me to enjoy the process of Kokoro 51 that I hadn't enjoyed in Kokoro 44. The first time around was about survival, the second time was an absolute blast!

Using the breathing technique I learned at Kokoro 44 allowed me to train harder and longer because I wasn't gassed out. Knowing how much running was required in the event, I ran more often and for longer distances. I also increased the overall volume of training, and continue to increase it for future events. You can never be too prepared.

I didn't always love training or pushing myself through major discomfort. Now it provides a huge feeling of accomplishment. I have the privilege of coaching several people who were much like me when I began this health and fitness journey. I love to watch them grow and break through the perceived barriers that they have lived with for years. Once the barrier is broken the growth really begins. The fear subsides and the sky is the limit.

The way I see it, once the bar is raised, it can't come down. It keeps raising repeatedly.

> *Not ready to lace up your sneakers and walk around the block?* "Do it anyway!"

INSIGHTS:

1. Learn the rules before you break them
2. Train in tough environments
3. Surround yourself with a team of people who share the same goal and they will never let you quit

CHAPTER 10

GORUCK SELECTION 021, PART 1

GORUCK Selection is modelled after Special Forces Selection. The cadre or coaches are active duty and retired Army Green Berets, Rangers, SEALs, and US Marine recon soldiers. The forty-eight-hour Selection is a condensed version of what they experience on the way to becoming Special Forces soldiers. They say it's every bit as challenging, just a shorter duration.

To prepare myself for this event I trained with coach Brad McCleod, Navy SEAL-retired, CEO of Seal Grinder PT, and a heck of a nice guy. Each week he would send workouts which were to be completed once or twice daily. I would follow his instructions and combine them with my own programming as I knew what my weaknesses were and what I needed to work on.

I wasn't a great runner, but I could do five miles in under forty minutes, consistently. However, I needed to make sure that I could be well under the mark with my nerves and everything else screaming during the event. One glaring weakness was the crab walk with a backpack in my lap. It's especially strenuous on the wrists. Another tough one was low crawling on my belly with a pack on or laying on my back with my feet six inches off the deck doing flutter kicks. I worked on mobility, adding additional yoga classes, and spent more time sitting in the bottom of the squat with a heavy pack overhead — I focused on the things that I had seen in previous candidates' experiences.

If you haven't practiced the exercises, it becomes very evident. Having watched the videos of previous Selections classes, I could see who received special attention and why. I specifically worked on the things that would come up in the welcome party. People who had poor mobility or had not worked on those things specifically, simply couldn't do them well and they'd get singled out by the cadre and pulled off to the side, worked on until they got it right or quit. I knew I had to work hard enough to be able to be in the middle of the pack, because I also knew that I was never going to be the strongest or the fastest in the group. But, with proper training, I could stay in the middle until I wasn't in the middle anymore!

If I could go back in time, back to my twenties, I would sign up to enter the Special Forces. I have endless respect for the sacrifices that these people have made and the commitment to serving their country and fellow man. It is a service-oriented job. Whatever I used to believe it was, or imagined it was like, doesn't come close to the reality of the job. Much like doctors who have completed many tiers of education to obtain specialized skills to serve mankind, Special Forces require equal education and preparation. They are selfless beings. It's a very humbling experience to have the honor to learn from them and be in their presence. That's one of the main reasons I keep going back; I learn so much.

My GORUCK Selection experience started at 12:30 on Thursday afternoon, October 17, 2019 in Jacksonville, Florida. We had received an email the day before telling us the exact location of the event. After receiving the email I scouted the location to make sure I knew where it was. It was a peaceful park just off the beach. The next day I took an Uber to the event and spotted the GORUCK tent setup as we arrived. I decided to hang back for a while and avoid being the first one rushing to sign in. Once everybody started to file in, I approached the tent, sensing and observing the tension in the participants, myself included.

In an attempt to maintain a level of calmness, I sat down next to my ruck and just watched what was going on. Did a little stretching and drank water in order to maintain hydration. It was already about 80° F and humid. We were told to stand up and check in. We each received a roster number based on the order that we registered. Mine was 012. Out of the 224 candidates who had signed up ahead and paid their money, only fifty-nine actually showed up. Out of those, only three finished.

The first order of business was the ruck weigh-in. The minimum requirement is forty-five pounds dry, before any food or water is added. I had weighed it myself beforehand and knew it was forty-seven pounds.

When I placed my ruck on the scales the numbers fluctuated and finally settled on 45.5. My scales at home must have been off. Luckily, I was still in. I had a three-quart bladder inside my ruck and also two military 'Meals Ready to Eat', some snacks plus oral rehydration salts. They are essentially the same formula administered by IV at a hospital if required. They dissolve in one liter of water and consumed as required. I always had one of them at the ready in a Nalgene bottle in addition to the water in the bladder, determined to not get dehydrated.

We lined up in silence, as we were not allowed to speak. Once checked in, the rules apply and if you speak to another candidate it's called an integrity violation and you are sent home. We stood there longer than necessary. Enough time to question ourselves about our desire to be there. Like Kokoro, this is by design to start adding mental pressure. And it works — well!

The standards for Selection are as follows: You must be able to complete a minimum of fifty-five push-ups in two minutes, sixty-five sit-ups in two minutes. Run five miles in under forty minutes and ruck twelve miles in three hours thirty minutes or less while wearing your pack, containing forty-five pounds minimum, dry. Meaning before any consumables or water were added.

As we waited to perform the first part of the test, we stood in six rows with our backs to the candidates that were undergoing the test.

First were the fifty-five push-ups in a two-minute period without stopping. We were allowed to rest with our hips in the air or in a bowed position, like a yoga pose, as long as our knees or our body did not touch the ground. I know my pace and how many push-ups I can do. Typically, I can do a minimum of sixty-five in two minutes. It was my turn and I was on a slight slope positioned with my feet higher than my hands. Cadre Ricky was counting the push-ups while he held onto the sheet with my roster number, medical details, and personal info.

I was doing push-ups and had completed whatever number it was when cadre Mocha called out, "One minute." I took a short rest and kept going. At that point, I was feeling great; up and down, up and down, it was easy. Cadre Ricky said, "Lower." Then added, "If I'm talking to you, I'm not counting the rep." There were a few times when he told me that I needed to go either higher or lower. He was not counting out loud so I didn't know exactly where I was at.

On the push-up that I thought was fifty-four, I stalled. I was at the bottom pushing myself up and I was shaking all over. I thought to myself, "Oh my god! No, no, no! I'm not going to fail out of this thing in the first —" He called, "Time." I fell flat on my chest and then got up quickly to see what Cadre Ricky had to say. He turned the sheet toward me: it was fifty-five. To myself, I thought, "Thank frickin' goodness!" I was still in. With the combined pressure of nerves, heat, tension, and the slope, it wasn't as easy as I anticipated. I thought I had a huge buffer, especially because push-ups are my strongest movement when it comes to body weight PT, and yet I barely made it.

We returned to the line and waited until it was time for the sit-ups. I could barely reach sixty-five most times, so I started mentally prepping myself, saying, "Okay, I have this timed out. I have to just do them at the pace that I know I can, just to get to sixty-five." I had cadre Ricky again, and I noticed again that there was a tiny bit of a slope, this time in a more favorable direction as my feet were slightly lower than my hips. Someone held my feet, and off I went; I banged out seventy-two, which was my personal best. I thought, "Okay. Awesome. This is great. I got this!" And my optimism was renewed.

A handful of people didn't meet the standards and had to retest. And even then, only some of them made it. I really felt for the participants that had flown all the way there with all their gear, booked a hotel and a rental car, only to be sent home within a couple of hours because they couldn't do the push-ups or sit-ups.

After the event, I spoke with a couple of them and they said, "I could bang out this many…." But as I've said before, it's an entirely different ballgame when it's in your own gym with the music cranked and you're fresh. It's very different trying to do them when you haven't slept very well the night before because of your nerves, the heat, the stress — all of these are major contributing factors.

Once the remaining candidates had passed the push-ups and sit-ups, or were sent home, we ruck-marched to the beach. We took off the packs and headed out to the hard-packed sand where we immediately ran five miles up and down the beach.

We ran straight into the wind on the way there. I'm an adequate runner, but at fifty-three I was the oldest candidate and was feeling a little challenged. There was a guy named Rob who was forty-six, but the rest all seemed to be in their twenties and thirties. I made a mental note not to use my age as an excuse.

At the turnaround point, I was second last. I started thinking, "Uh oh, this isn't good." But when I turned around, I began running better as the wind was at my back. I played a mental game with myself where I would see a guy up ahead and say, "Okay, that guy." And I would run until I passed him then, "That guy. Okay. Now that woman. I'm going to chase her down until I pass her." I passed about six or seven people this way and completed the challenge with less than two minutes to spare. (38:24.) Only one person did not make the time due to an ankle sprain. The fastest person finished at sub-thirty-five minutes — I was incredibly impressed with his time.

The way they had it setup in previous Selection classes, they did the push-ups, sit-ups, followed by the five-mile run. Once the run was complete, you have a bit of time to change into your pants, boots, and make sure your water bladder is topped up. Then it would be time for the twelve-mile ruck. Little did we know they were about to change this up on us....

When we arrived at our gear after running; the cadre told us, "You've got about ten minutes to take care of priorities of work." I managed to pull my pants on quick enough, took my running shoes off and put them in my pack. I had just pulled my right boot on when the cadre came at us, screaming: "Get your rucks on and low crawl to the ocean now!"

I had one boot in my hand and no sock on my left foot. I put my ruck on, started belly crawling and continued trying to pull my sock on, which at this point was filled with sand. Obviously, my foot was full of sand and I tried to dust it off but the cadre came at me again screaming to just do it on the run. "What if you were getting shot at in combat? Would you stop to put your boot on? No!" Move!

Somehow, I slipped my boot on while crawling along but it came at the price of being second last. Whoever was behind me was just getting reamed. I low crawled as fast as I could. I had practiced this movement often, minus the added pressure of the absent shoe of course! Despite that, it felt good to be able to catch up. The added motivation of a little fear and adrenaline pumping didn't hurt. I managed to gain ground and get into the middle to upper part of the pack by the time we got to the ocean. Once we made it to the ocean, they instantly had us do burpees with our backpacks on — forty-five, fifty, sixty pounds — whatever they weighed at that point. It was up and down, up and down, followed by crawling, and bear crawling.

Once the rinse in the ocean was done, I mentally prepped myself for the upcoming hike. "On your feet and fall in," instructed a cadre. We hiked back to the checkpoint where we started a few short hours before and I thought, "Alright, now the hike's going to start." But like I said, they were about to switch things up on our group. Just as we arrived, Cadre Jason had us march past the check-in tent, to an open culvert about four or five feet wide and about 100 yards long. It contained several inches of mud and goose shit. He told us all to head to the end of the ditch and low crawl all the way back. Rucks on.

We were on our bellies low crawling and he yelled, "Get muddy. I don't want to see any bare skin." Of course, we were already completely covered from head to toe, backpacks full too. There was a low bridge that we had to crawl under, so I took my pack off, and pushed it through while low crawling, then put it back on. Some people just said, "Enough of this," stood up, and just bailed.

When we got through, it was time to stand up and fall into formation with the weight of the pack heavier than ever, and although we're not allowed to smile, on the inside I was smiling ear to ear. I thought, "Oh my god, this is so much fun!" This shift in mindset is the result of all the training. There's a saying that Special Forces use called, "Embrace the suck". You can fight it and complain to yourself, have a negative mindset, or you can embrace it, wholeheartedly, and enjoy it. It's a choice.

I can feel like this is fun because I know that I can handle it. I know I've gotten to a point where this is really hard, it really hurts, but it's not going to get any worse. I can take it and this will pass. It was yet another perceived barrier that I pushed through.

Next we began running through residential areas. Cadre Jason ran behind us holding a cell phone while he commentated on a Facebook Live feed and said, "Man, I wouldn't want to be at the back. I hate last place. It pays to be a winner."

It's the truth; you really don't want to be in the back. It was like a leapfrog race with about forty people racing to get up to the front. I paced myself and tried to plan it out strategically. I figured, "All right. I'm almost at the back. Now it's time to run around these people and get to the front." This went on for an incalculable amount of time.

Finally, we reached the swamp where there was a huge pile of sand on a tarp and a stack of empty sandbags. We were then tasked with filling every empty sandbag that we could see. "You've got three minutes." We jumped into action and filled them as fast as we could. "We don't want to see a grain of sand left. That tarp needs to be folded up and handed to us when you're done."

Of course, we can never meet their time hacks because we're not supposed to. At a certain point they yelled, "Drop the sandbags!" and ordered us to line up. Next, we started doing these insane exercises. Overhead carries with the ruck, overhead squats, and then we were told to put our rucks on. Next it was time to play a game the cadre call 'little man in the woods.' The rules of the game are, while wearing your backpack, you must slowly lower yourself into a squat and then back up again all the while performing jumping jacks. It was one of the most arduous things I had ever done. This went on for what felt like eternity.

We played that game until the cadre decided it was enough. Then it was back to filling the sandbags. Again they gave some arbitrary time, "Okay. You've got 'this' long." Followed by, "No, you didn't meet it. Back in formation." More of the 'little man in the fucking woods'! They piled on more ruck PT, burpees, and whatever they could come up with to make it as strenuous as possible.

Finally, on the third round, we got it all. We had filled every sandbag and folded the tarp; some of them weighed 60 pounds but most of them weighed 80 pounds or more. We were then divided into two groups, a Northern Group and a Southern Group. The next iteration began. I was in the Southern Group and we each had to carry a sandbag on top of our rucks while carrying a lit tiki torch. We looked like we were walking to tribal council in an episode of *Survivor* as we walked along a narrow path next to the swamp. We spaced out the torches out as directed by the cadre in order to provide light for our next exercise. The torches emitted a lot of smoke — it was like training at a truck stop.

We were told to run to the end of the road, and bear crawl back. Run to the end and low crawl back. Then run and crab walk back, followed by lunges. My friends and family told me afterward, "We only saw you once on camera." I explained, "Yeah, that's by design. If you're on camera early on, it's because you're in the back of the pack, and you've been singled out."

The crab walk was the one I had the toughest time with. There was only one guy behind me, and the rest of the pack was ahead, although not by much. Nonetheless, Jason came up with the camera in my face, and said, "That guy is last. He's going to quit soon. That's going to make you last. I'm coming back," then he added, "And you don't want to be last." I scooted up as far as I could, just to stay off of his radar.

We did 200 meters each of crab walk, bear crawls, etc. Next we had to choose a sandbag and follow the cadre. Something I learned from one of the guys who finished was how important it was to conserve energy. The guy was a master at it. This was his fourth time attempting Selection, and although he made it to the top three in previous Selection classes, he had not made it to the end. I found myself keeping an eye on him to see what he was doing and followed along.

I was under the impression we had to do everything perfectly, but that's not the case. We merely need to put in our best effort, especially when the cadre are watching. As long as I was doing the exercise to meet the standard they'd leave me alone. If anyone did not keep up with the standard, they'd stay on them, keep hounding them and eventually the participant would quit because physically, it's just too much.

On top of the fifty- to sixty-pound ruck on our backs, we had an eighty-pound sandbag that we had to carry to the next cadre. Each cadre we would arrive at would give us a new exercise, like suitcase carry it in one hand, or drag it. Sometimes we had to front carry it, which is like carrying an eighty-pound baby in your arms. All, while trying to keep your elbows up! Or we'd have to overhead carry it, or carry it on one shoulder then switch it to the other shoulder as we walked.

It didn't take long to figure out which ones were the toughest to do. As soon as I'd be up and around the bend a little, out of the cadre's line of sight, I'd start dragging it. We'd take advantage of any kind of little trick that we could use to conserve energy. The cadre know about these hacks; they're not stupid. They went through this as well, but we'd gain ground when we could, and we'd adhere strictly to the standards when we absolutely had to.

As the exercises continued, I realized this was still "the welcome party." At all of the previous Selection events that I had researched the welcome party was the four-hour beat down that was administered after the twelve-mile ruck. Our welcome party lasted eight hours! The speed, the intensity, and the duration we were subjected to, was far greater than anything I had anticipated.

Kokoro was very intense and it was hot but it was manageable. Selection consisted of everything that we had to do at Kokoro, but with a sixty-pound rucksack on our backs and with no breaks. It was a constant barrage, it was like Kokoro on steroids. Prior to Selection I messaged someone that I knew had completed Kokoro and had also attended Selection. I asked "How much harder is Selection than Kokoro?" He simply replied, "It's harder." That's all he said. I wanted to know more, "Oh thanks, buddy. How much harder?" No words can explain how tough it is, which he knew. I found that out on my own. The way everyone should.

At Kokoro, as I've mentioned, the cadre were not trying to make us quit; they wanted us to be challenged, but not quit. At Selection, they really pushed us to what seemed impossible for the majority. It's simply the standard that has to be upheld, and they aren't going to abandon it for anybody. Many of the participants at Selection were close, personal friends of the cadre. Yet they do not lower the standards for friend or foe. It is a horribly fair event.

Many of those who have successfully completed Selection come back to watch and support. I had the opportunity to meet a few of them and chat for a bit after the event. Just realizing what it took for them to finish is more than inspiring, but it's also understanding just how difficult it truly is.

When we finally finished strolling down tiki lane with our sandbags we marched over to a small enclosed field which was surrounded by palm trees. It had a huge bonfire burning directly in the center. The swamp was on the other side of the trees. "Okay. Now we're going to play America's favorite pastime. We're going to play baseball; cadre baseball."

Of course, I had no idea what that was, but it sounded like it was going to be hard. They had a large Home Depot bucket with a bunch of cards in it. The cards read things like, "First base: twenty-five push-ups. Second base: twenty burpees. Third base: fifteen eight-count body builders. Right field: Clean and jerk with a sandbag. Center field: Squat. Left field: Dead lifts." All movements to be performed with an eighty-pound sandbag. Of course, all while wearing our rucksacks. If we hit a home run, we had to run to first base, bear crawl to second base, crab walk to third, and run home.

This went on for many, many hours and was actually my favorite part of my time at Selection; it was a blast. The main reason I enjoyed it so much was that if I just kept working, the cadre left me alone. It was manageable. We could game it a little bit here and there, maybe shave a few reps here and there. Or we'd look at our card, and hand it to the cadre who would then tell us, "Okay. Home run." By the time the next person came up, he'd be distracted. I would tell myself, "Screw that. I'm not doing a home run. I'm going to go to dead lift," and I'd work my way around it. We were at it for hours, but at least messing with the rules helped a little. Burpees were good for this, because as long as we kept moving, they wouldn't call you out on it. We'd drop down slowly, kind of pop back up, do a little hop and continue along like that. Again, the cadre are well aware of the tricks but it really doesn't matter. The amount of work that a candidate has to do to be able to finish Selection is unfathomable. Shaving a few reps may buy a little time but eventually the mental game is what counts. The people that finish Selection finish due to mental strength. Everyone's body is beat to shit. Like cadre Jason says "It's just work doin' the work".

I remember doing push-ups when a cadre came over to me and said, "Look, if you keep moving, I'll leave you alone. If you're going to just lay there, I'm coming back." I took that as a very good hint to just put more effort in, and that's what I did.

There were several people who were vomiting due to dehydration. One of them was a woman who had attempted Selection several times before and was a good friend of Jason's. She became dehydrated and I believe it had happened to her two or three other times, so perhaps it's a medical issue, but at that point she left.

The cadre say some funny shit. It was always eerily quiet; we weren't even allowed to grunt and groan. The cadre would say, "No sex noises," or, "Suffer in silence!" I could hear the cadre moving from candidate to candidate, saying things that were just hilarious but of course we couldn't laugh or even react. I remember at some point somebody was in the swamp and the cadre was kicking water at him saying, "Don't drink the water. You're not a fish." When you're in the heat of the moment, these things are quite funny.

Cadre baseball finished and cadre Jason (CEO of GORUCK), said, "Normally you don't get any food for the first twenty-four hours, but you guys have been working so hard, we're going to give you a snack." I've never seen such a feeding frenzy! Everybody was running over each other, tripping and falling, because we thought that maybe there wasn't enough for everybody. We all managed our allotted share of one banana and one granola bar.

For the next part, we had to take our rucksacks off and hold them overhead while standing in formation. Jason said, "All right. We're just going to do this until somebody quits." We held them up above our heads for who knows how long. I let my ruck rest on my head for a moment until I heard, "Hey old man, get that ruck off of your head." I turned to look at him. "You know who I am talking to." Like I said… funny shit. The moment somebody dropped out he said, "Okay. Rucks down." Then we laid on our backs, holding our ruck in front of us just above our chests doing four count flutter kicks, which are like scissor kicks. One, two, three, one. One, two, three, two… Then, once somebody quit it was, "On your feet. Rucks overhead, find the bottom of the squat." We lifted the ruck overhead, then sunk into a deep squat and held it. Thanks to yoga my mobility is quite good, so it wasn't an issue. I was able to drop down and sit there and wait until somebody quit. Another dropped.

Finally came the twelve-mile hike, or what we thought was a twelve-mile hike. The cadre did not tell us if it was timed, or if it was a 'go' or 'no-go', as they say. 'Go' means you passed. 'No-go' means you're out. As alluded to earlier, the twelve-mile ruck is a standard that you have to be able to meet in order to keep going, and you need to finish it in under three hours thirty minutes.

We were told to walk 800 meters to a turnaround point where another set of cadre were waiting. They had our roster numbers on a list and would check us off each time we made it to a checkpoint. Back and forth we'd go along the dirt road next to the swamp.

Since we all thought it was a timed twelve-mile ruck march, many participants were running. I know what my pace is and I can do twelve miles in under three hours no problem. I have a long stride. I focused on my breathing and hydration and went for a leisurely hike. To me it was manageable and I thought it would be a piece of cake. I couldn't have been more wrong.

> *Do you feel like you aren't ready to sign up for a challenge?* "Do it anyway!"

INSIGHTS:

1. Visualize your desired outcome
2. Do a dry run to prepare for the real thing
3. Calm your nerves by controlling your breathing
4. Working out in an air-conditioned gym with your favorite tunes blaring doesn't prepare you for the real world

5. Embrace the suck
6. Doing the work is less difficult than observing what needs to be done
7. You have to help yourself before you can help others

CHAPTER 11

GORUCK SELECTION 021, PART 2

It was a beautiful night even though it was cool by Florida standards in October; it was about fifty degrees. When we stopped moving, it could feel a little chilly. I was soaking wet and the cold was sinking in. I couldn't stop to urinate every time I needed to or I'd have been stopping continuously. I was careful to avoid dehydration, which could induce vomiting, and ultimately lead to being dropped for medical reasons. I was more than likely over-cautious and probably drank more than I should have. As a result, I was literally peeing in my pants as we rucked from checkpoint to checkpoint. Luckily, there are drain holes in my Nike SF jungle boots.

Reading this you're likely thinking that's disgusting. But when you're in the moment and it's pass or fail, urine-saturated pants and boots are not a concern. At approximately mile ten I began to notice that I was badly chafing. Sand and mud had become lodged in my groin and under the ruck straps. Trapped there while low-crawling in the culvert. I wore GORUCK Challenge pants. They are lightweight and very durable. Fantastic pants. It is highly "recommended" that you "go commando" to allow the mud and sand to exit and avoid chafing. Of course, I ignored this and wore shorts underneath. The sand was there to stay and I was chafing with every step. More than a little uncomfortable. After about three hours of continuous hiking, cadre Mocha said, "Okay. That's twelve miles. Just keep walking until one of the cadre tell you to stop."

Roger that. I was feeling great, apart from the chafing. I felt strong and ready for anything. It was a dark night and completely silent. The only illumination came from the occasional glimpse of the moon and the Chem lights on the backs of our rucks. I was able to pass some people as I had the twelve-mile pace dialed in, while others lapped me as they ran by. Turns out it did not matter, since it wasn't a go or no-go situation. Soon after the completion of mile 15 I ran out of water.

I headed over to the truck where Cadre Mocha Mike sat monitoring our progress. Cadre Mocha (named after his love of café mocha) is infamous in the GORUCK community. He has been with the company for many years and he's an awesome guy. The cadre are as harsh as can be but they also have the biggest hearts. They want us to succeed, they're on our side all while trying to make us quit. It's a strange dynamic but if you have ever seen videos of past events, the cadre often speak about how much they are rooting for us. When they finish speaking to the camera they switch back to cadre mode to administer another set of harsh commands.

I approached the truck and called out to Mocha to let him know that I was black on water. He pointed me in the direction of where to fill up. My pack was full of mud and I wasn't able to adjust the straps up or down, which was entirely my own fault. The zippers felt like they were welded together which made it really tough to open and close in order to get the bladder out.

There was mud packed between my body and the ruck strap, chafing away every bit of skin it touched. Once I took the pack off, the stinging stopped for a moment, then I started to get cold. Once the bladder was full I realized how badly my groin was chafed.

What came next I can only call a miscalculation, a major mental error and it was almost like watching somebody else walk from my rucksack to the truck and say, "Hey, Cadre Mocha, I'm done!" He looked up at me and said, "Why? You look strong; why are you quitting?" He had no emotion in his voice having seen this countless times. Firmly, I elaborated just enough to remove any confusion, "I'm not putting that fucking ruck back on." Mike just looked at me and said, "Okay." Once those words were out of my mouth, I was officially done. No excuses.

Had this been at Kokoro the coaches would have tried to talk me through it with inspiring and motivating words. My teammates would have said, "Come on, man, we got you. You got this." Often that's all that would be needed to get through a weak moment.

We had no one working on us during the hike, no one yelling or trying to make us quit. This was when my mind started question why I was there. I started to psyche myself out. This evolution leaves you to your own thoughts, it is brilliant on their part; they know how we're going to react in that environment under those conditions. Once the quit door is open a crack it is just a matter of time... There must have been close to ten people that DOR (dropped on request) during the hike.

Once I quit, I went back to my pack, and started to feel the regret instantly, "What the fuck have I just done?" I questioned myself. I had so much left in the tank, but I let that mental lapse get to me, due to physical discomfort. Chafing and other types of irritations had happened before, why did I let it get in my head this time? Countless participants have endured far worse. I had forgotten my WHY. Lesson learned.

I limped over to the quitters fire and warmed up with the others that had dropped out. When the evolution ended a few minutes later there were fifteen participants left out of the fifty-nine that began.

They ran past us for more PT, burpees, and other methods of torture that the cadre prescribed. Nothing that they weren't used to. Not long after that they were in the swamp. They came out with clean rucks and their bodies were free of mud and sand. I would have been able to remove some of the sand and mud in my groin and carried on. Who knows for how long? Coulda, shoulda, woulda. All bullshit. It was completely my fault due to mental weakness and poor gear execution.

Thinking back, I remember how nice the night was. I strolled along, barely feeling the weight of the ruck. The swamp was illuminated by the light of the moon, the air was crisp and clear, and all I could hear was my steady breathing and the occasional footsteps of another participant. If it wasn't for the pain in my muscles and the mud in my groin, I could have fooled myself into thinking it was a nighttime walk in the park. We were just walking back and forth, back and forth, and I felt a million bucks. I was thanking God and thinking about friends and family back home and about how certain I was that I had a great shot at finishing Selection. I felt awesome. "It's been hard, but I'm managing." I said to myself, "Yeah, I got this." The mental shift was abrupt and came without warning.

When I had stopped to fill the bladder in my ruck, the zippers in the ruck barely opened or closed. Of course, I hadn't rinsed them off like the other guys had told me to do. "Use your water bottle to rinse the mud out of your zippers and clean the straps so they can slide." The little tricks that they knew through experience which I didn't until it was too late. I went from feeling awesome and saying, "I'm going to finish this thing," to, "That's it, I'm done," a split-second decision full of regret. But I learned from it, and I won't make that mistake again.

It was definitely fun despite being so difficult. This type of event is more difficult to watch and think about than it is to actually participate in. Opinions may vary. It looks more difficult than it actually is, if you've done the appropriate training. If you're not fit enough, it is too daunting.

I think that's probably applicable in some ways to many things in life. When you take a step back and look at things from a distance, your brain can run wild coming up with potential scenarios. But once you're in it, you have no choice but to deal with it and to go through it. You prepare as best as you can. I read somebody's AAR (After Action Report) in which they said, "Well, I guess you're never fully prepared. It's just like, how do you prepare for a kick in the nuts? You know it's coming, but it's still going to hurt like heck."

I really beat myself up after quitting because I fully expected to be able to get through. Since I had completed both Kokoro events and the second one was much harder. I had trained even harder for Selection. I thought I was physically and mentally prepared for it. I fully admit that I was not prepared enough. My mental game must improve prior to next

Selection. Yes, there will be a next time. I will be a year or two older and hopefully a little wiser.

I felt better just knowing that very few people complete it the first try. Most people require several attempts. There are many important things to learn. How and when to conserve energy and as well as gear tips and tricks. Something as simple as zipper lubrication can save much needed time and aggravation. Chafing is inevitable but you can control the severity if managed properly.

We signed waivers at the start of Selection, acknowledging that we could sustain serious injury and possibly die. We were responsible to advise the cadre if we felt ill or if we had vomited.

Injury, illness, and death are rare in the ultra-endurance community but they do occur. There are people who have died of hyponatremia during Special Forces training, a condition caused by drinking too much water, but not having enough electrolytes or salts in the body to absorb it. Both GORUCK Selection and SEALFIT Kokoro events had medics present. They were well identified and on constant watch. We repeatedly heard, "Safety first." The cadre want everyone to get the most from the experience. Ultimately, these events are designed to help us grow as human beings. It's all about growth. As cadre Jason says "The human spirit is alive and well."

The difference between the two events is that Selection is based on the standards of becoming a Special Forces soldier, where they are actively trying to make us quit. Whereas, although Kokoro is extremely difficult, the focus is on teamwork and leadership, not trying to make the candidates quit. The cadre could certainly do this if they wanted to; the purpose reflects the methodology.

During Selection, I found myself wanting to help other candidates at certain points, the way I had done at Kokoro, but then I had to remind myself, "No. I'm not here to do that. The less of that I do, the closer I am to finishing." I frequently had to flip my thoughts to suit the purpose of the event. One minute I realized it's an intense competition, hoping others would quit, then wanting to lend a hand or an occasional "You got this". You must have laser focus with the end goal in mind. This is one occasion where "nice guys really do finish last".

Huge respect and congratulations to the three warriors that completed Selection 021:
- Patrick Mies AKA Ruck Jesus (roster #008)
- Alex Kaliniak AKA Peanut Butter (roster #051)
- Mark Jones (roster #042)

> *Rather watch than participate?* "Do it anyway!"

INSIGHTS:

1. Set micro goals when things get really difficult
2. Start! Put your running shoes on, step outside, walk to the corner, then to the next corner
3. Do one more rep
4. Drink one more glass of water
5. Sign up for something, anything, and train for it
6. Micro goals add up

CHAPTER 12

THINGS I'VE LEARNED

If I could go back and talk to my younger self, the biggest message I would try to hammer home is, "You're good enough. You belong here. You've earned it, and you're good enough to stay. Put in the effort, and you'll be fine. Don't quit. Don't bail when it gets tough. Don't sell yourself short and don't look for the easy route because it doesn't promote growth." It took a while for me to get there but after accomplishing these goals and challenges, I proved to myself that I can really do anything if I put the effort in. For me, it started with physical fitness goals; perseverance to push past the limits where the discomfort started and where the natural ability ended. We're not all of a sudden mentally tough. Maybe some people are, depending how they're brought up and their life experience, but I don't think most people are. I certainly wasn't. I gained it by reading books like *Unbeatable Mind* and *The Way of the SEAL*, both by Mark Divine, David Goggins' book *You Can't Hurt Me* and many other books that taught me how to use the tools. There are so many tools available to use in order to achieve mental toughness.

The first tool I found to push my physical limits was to do one more repetition, or five more or whatever the next number was that I thought I couldn't do. That helped me stop putting a limit on myself and my capabilities. As written by Rob Roy and Chris Lawson in their book *The Navy SEAL Art of War*: "Ask the average man on the street how many push-ups he can do and you will likely get a straight answer. While striving to be honest and, at the same time, burnish his ego, he'll say something like 'I can do twenty-five' or 'I can knock out forty.' A straight shooter. Ask that same question to a SEAL and you will get a much different response. 'I can do at least one hundred.' And therein lies the ethos of a SEAL — we think in terms of possibilities, not limitations."

I started by telling myself, "Okay. One more. One more. Okay, I'm going to stop when I get to this number. No, I'm not going to stop when I get to that number. And so on. Continually pushing to the next level, past the previous limit.

It is akin to a mental muscle, expanding, pushing the line a little bit further and a little bit further each time. Very soon that line is a long way away from the line where you started, and you have that much more mental strength.

I also see it in the clients I train when they say, "Wow, I had no idea that I could do that!" after completing a twelve-hour crucible. We don't know what we're capable of until we push past the limits, which are really just *perceived* limits.

When a sprinter is running a race, she doesn't slow down when she sees the finishing line. She speeds up. She doesn't quit running when someone passes her, she runs faster. When she sees the finishing line, she doesn't aim for it, she aims for a spot beyond it. To aim for the finishing line and slow down just as you're nearing it, is equal to going through life only giving eighty percent. In your mind, you need to be that sprinter.

One of the teachings that stands out from my time with Mark Divine was, "When you think you're finished doing whatever physical activity you're doing, you're only forty percent of the way there. You've got another sixty percent in the tank." It's only our minds that hold us back. The body says, "Man, I've got lots left. Let's go." But the mind says, "Oh, that's enough." Turn off the governor.

Once I was able to push past the first barrier, then the second, the third, the fourth, and so on… I learned to thrive on it. In the beginning I thought: "Whoa man, this is hard. I better slow down and stop." But once I knew that there's no limit, or the limit was further away than I thought it was, I just kept pushing myself harder. I still do.

That's not to say that I don't still wrestle with limitations, or the feeling of 'not being enough.' I still struggle with it today, however not when it comes to physical training or these events, it's in other areas, like a relationship, an audition, or public speaking that I need to keep working. Even while writing this book I'm thinking, "Why would anyone want to know about my life? What's so great about it?" But I realize that these lessons can potentially help people.

That feeling of not being good enough was different as a parent raising my kids. Kids observe everything; it's not just what you say to them, it's your actions. My daughter was the first person I spoke to when I finished Kokoro. All three kids were watching via Instagram posts, and would make comments throughout. Initially it wasn't on Facebook Live as it is now. She called and said, "I'm so proud of you. That's so awesome.

I'm so happy you did this." That was my biggest "WHY" for doing Kokoro; to be an example for my kids, to show them if you put your mind to it and push yourself, you can accomplish it. There was absolutely no way I could quit.

My "WHY", or my reasons, for doing Selection were as follows (they may change for the next one):

To be an example for older athletes. That they too can take control of their minds and bodies, and their spirit will follow. Get off the couch and take charge of their health. If I can, they can.

We live in a weak society and I want to inspire people to take the hard road, not the easy path. Grow, change, challenge.

Push through my fear boundaries. Fear of people, success, public speaking, and auditions.

I am too old for Special Forces but I want to prove that I could have made it. Perhaps, that's my ego wanting it, but it was a motivator.

To become a better father, leader, role model, actor and coach.

To find out what I am truly capable of and to solidify a never-quit attitude.

Some people need additional support. There is absolutely no shame in seeking therapy if that's the road that somebody needs to take. We all have things from our past, maybe stemming from childhood, that shaped us, scarred us, and sometimes professional help might need to be added to mix.

If somebody is dealing with addictions, be it food, alcohol, drugs, sex, gambling, cell phones, social media or whatever it may be, there are many support programs available that can help with them. I'm not going to name them, but they're easy to find. Feel free to get in touch with me and I will gladly help you source the support that you need. We are never alone.

If your health has gone by the wayside because you haven't focused on it, put a focus on just getting started. That's all — it just takes starting. There are so many fitness coaches, gurus and nutritionists available, pick one and start. It doesn't matter who it is, if one doesn't work out, go to the next one until the right fit occurs.

Just get off the couch and start moving your body. Maybe it's simply walking around the block in the beginning. Next week, maybe it's a jog, and then maybe you're able to run, or get into the gym and move. If you don't know what to do, start light with body weight movements and get going. You'll begin to feel better. Over time, when you get to that twenty minutes plus spot where the endorphins kick in, serotonin will release, and if you can be out in nature, it is going to help with your mood tremendously.

There are people who suffer from depression, and other mental and emotional challenges that may require medication or a doctor's supervision. If you need it, seek it. Don't take my life insights as a replacement for a doctor's advice. However, if you can feel better after you exercise, then that's a good thing. Continue! I found as I started to train, I ate better. The desire for crappy food diminished the more fit I became and the more focus I put on getting fit. I'm not a nutritionist and I don't advise people on how to eat. There are many nutritionists out there and at least as many different diets. Trying to navigate them all and keep up with the latest trends is nearly impossible. There seems to be new diets popping up every year. I experimented with many of them until I figured out what works best for me. Get educated on the subject and figure out what's best for you. And if you want to save some time, find a professional that resonates with your beliefs.

Once the first steps are taken you'll begin to feel better and insulin sensitivity may improve as you lose a few pounds. Fitness, like many areas of life, requires momentum. Like trying to roll a boulder. Once you start moving and gain some momentum, it continues. One of my rules, especially in the beginning, is never take more than one day off in a row.

I'm not a believer in New Year's resolutions and I do not make them. I have learned to map out a plan when I need to change something. I find out how to do it and go for it. Fitness is not a goal for me. It is a way of life. If you can get to the point where it becomes a way of life, it's a whole lot easier than setting a weight loss target.

Yes, smaller goals are awesome. If you want to get into that pair of pants, perfect. Maybe you want to look better in a swimsuit, or you want to go to a specific event, they're all great stepping stones and temporary targets, but they're not the end goal.

I don't have body composition goals. Body composition happens as *the* result of training. Health is the goal. It was only a few months ago that I went to get my blood work tested, just to see where I was with my testosterone levels. At the same time, they checked cholesterol, blood sugar and a variety of standard markers. All came back with flying colors. That wasn't the case in my twenties when my cholesterol levels were through the roof. I was in trouble and the first thing the doctor asked me was, "How much do you drink?" I said, "I don't know, like a couple of beers a week, here and there not much." She could tell I was lying through my teeth.

Having optimal health and fitness is how I want to live in my older years. What do I want my quality of life to be? Fitness needs to be my way of life; not a short-term goal, not a fad diet or workout like a crazy person for a month just to get into a swimsuit then stop.

Look in the mirror and ask yourself if you are happy with your current level of health? This is not about your hair color, or your clothing. Are you happy with how you see yourself? Are you happy with how you feel? It's not about other people's ideals; it's about your own.

Maybe you feel a few pounds overweight and less attractive than you used to? Are you happy with the state of your health? Can you do all the things that you want? Can you play a game of pick-up soccer with friends? Can you pick up your grandkids? Can you chase them around? If I said to you, "Tomorrow, we're going to go hike up a mountain with some weight in our packs; it's going to be three hours of fun and fitness! There's an unbelievable waterfall on the way and an amazing view from the top. Are you ready?" Could you do it? Or would the excuses begin to fly?

If you are fit enough, then let's go. Nothing can stop us. I had a client who used to say to me, "Man, I couldn't even walk a block. If the place I was headed to didn't have an elevator I wouldn't go." Is that anyway to live your life? Thankfully they changed their situation. Sure, that might be an extreme example, but what if somebody invited you to go play Frisbee golf, soccer, or go for a swim? Would you feel physically capable?

If you are extremely out of shape, the odds are there are going to be excuses as to why you can't participate in whatever the physical activity might be. We are never too far gone to make a start. When you're fit enough, all the possibilities open up. When we have a minimum level of physical fitness, the options available to us are huge. Then we truly have the choice to say no, instead of endless excuses.

Part of it comes down to taking ownership of your current physical state. Where are you at health and fitness-wise. Another fantastic book that I read is called *Extreme Ownership* by Jocko Willink and Leif Babin, both retired SEALs. Wherever I'm at, good or bad, it is my responsibility.

Oftentimes I think we get used to making excuses for everything without even noticing. I can remember back when I was 15 years old. I was the quarterback, playing football for the Sherwood Park Rams. I don't remember the coach's name but he was a Coca-Cola addict. One after the other; I can't recall ever seeing him without one in his hand. One time we were playing against Spruce Grove, a team that was always undefeated, and during the game, I remember rolling to the left during a passing play, I threw the ball, missed our receiver, and the other team intercepted it and ran for a touchdown. My coach was livid. He marched right up to me and the first thing I did was make an excuse. He grabbed my face mask and yelled at me nose-to-nose, "Excuses are for losers!"

I have never forgotten that, but all it did at the time was crush my self-esteem. If somebody said that to me now, I'd say, "Yes, you're fucking right." I will own it and work on changing the behavior. This is the difference in my attitude now as compared to the past. I can turn a negative into a positive. All credit goes to others for this fact. None of it was my doing. Making excuses chips away at our mental health, and chips away at self-esteem.

This is why my motto is, "Do it anyway". If you don't want to train today, "Do it anyway". I don't want to do any number of things — it could be sending an email, cleaning the house, training, making that difficult phone call, having a difficult conversation with a loved one, but do it anyway.

That slogan can be used in all areas of our lives. Do I do it in every area in my life? Not always; not every time. It's certainly so much better than it used to be. The main constant "do it anyway" discipline is fitness; there is no option for me. I always "do it anyway", no matter what. Inspiration and motivation can be fleeting and depend upon circumstances. These are meaningless emotions if we have discipline.

> *Don't want to believe that you can?* "Do it anyway!"

CHAPTER 13

DO IT ANYWAY!

On the path to big changes are many small steps fueled by "Do It Anyway" moments. At first you may not recognize a "Do It Anyway" moment, but when you look back at the times that you pushed through a hard decision or beat laziness, you will realize there was such a moment that resulted in the action you needed to take.

I have had "Do It Anyway" moments throughout my journey even when I was not fully aware of them. One of the times I was in Thailand and wanted to get my scuba diving license, but it thoroughly terrified me. Partly, I didn't think I was smart enough to pass the test based on the classroom portion of the PADI certificate. I was pleasantly surprised — and relieved — to discover that I did extremely well on the exams. The other part of my issue was that I had a real fear of diving! Then came the moment when we all had to go into the water with the scuba gear on, submerge and breathe through the regulator. I kneeled down and looked across at my girlfriend who was just like a fish in water; she was simply loving it, and I was panicking, almost hyperventilating.

It might have been the competitive nature in me take over at that moment as I looked at her stay underwater. Part of me wanted to quit; I wanted to jump up and rip that regulator out of my mouth, but I stayed down there and overcame it, and the fear went away. I did it anyway and the reward was great.

We went out a little bit deeper and they showed us how to work on our buoyancy. At some point I too took to it like a fish in water. If I would have jumped up and bailed, like I had often done when things got difficult or uncomfortable, I probably never would have done it again. I would have made some excuse as to why I didn't want to dive anymore or that I hated it.

When I'm training, I say, "Do it anyway" to myself. If others are close by and can hear me they might be thinking, "Shut up, Harlow," but I'm saying it all the time. One of the things I use to keep me pushing forward when I'm training is an alter ego I have created. When I'm training in these events, I'm not called Scott, it's Harlow. My Kokoro t-shirt just had my last name on it. It's as if this badass dude is taking on these super strenuous, challenging crucibles; that's Harlow.

It's almost like flipping a switch and becoming my own personal superhero. As goofy as that sounds, I equate it to acting in a way. Every single person out there can connect to that; it's becoming a better, stronger version of myself, by choice. I think that I've had to reinvent myself to a certain extent. I've had to let go of so many things from my past, and when I think about it, the persona of Harlow is so much more than Scott was.

Once I had that epiphany, I thought, "Can I put that Harlow shirt on in any other areas of life that I find challenging or fearful?" Of course! I can put on the Harlow shirt and walk into an audition or get up in front of a group of people and tell my story, give a keynote at a public speaking event. Skydiving terrifies the crap out of me and yet I will put on my Harlow shirt and do it. It's on a list of fears that I plan to overcome.

Perhaps the Harlow persona is my own form of mental preparation for the various events. Pro athletes, or any type of athlete for that matter, prepare for a game, in a certain way. I remember when I played hockey, I had a specific order in which I put all my gear on. First it was pants, then the right skate, the left skate, shoulder pads, right elbow pad, left elbow pad, it wasn't a superstition, but a ritual of getting prepared mentally.

There were preparatory things I said to myself, even as I stepped onto the ice, and the first stretch — all those things were habitual. Perhaps my own personal superhero is a continuation of that and it's just another way of getting mentally prepared for these extreme events. Scott might not be able to handle this, but Harlow sure can.

I've seen a remarkable transformation in my brother since he started training three times a week. He has come such a long way with regard to his level of fitness, and his ability to push himself further each time he trains. As he's pushed himself harder and further, he's gained self-confidence in other areas of his life and how he handles himself. In business, the way he speaks now is different due to the level of confidence that he's gained.

There were several guys I met at Kokoro involved in a program called Wake up Warrior, they are all very successful business people who have gone through some difficult times. I know nothing about the program other than the guys rave about it. It sounds incredible. They often talked about not living small. These skills and challenges carry over into all areas of our lives.

Initially it pissed me off because I thought they were arrogant (they weren't). I watched how they were, but secretly I was envious of their level of confidence. I'm not serving myself or anyone else well by living small or being timid in any situation. When I started writing this book, I told myself this story was no big deal. I lived it; it's not that great! However, I was reminded everybody has done great things in their lives, and perhaps my transformation is a little more impressive than I think.

Part of that is humility. I want to have humility while not living small. There's a balance to be found between those two things.

The next time you find yourself ready to give up or failing to begin, remind yourself greatness awaits those that commit, so do it anyway!

> *If I can, you can.* "Do it anyway!"

EPILOGUE

It is September 2020, and we are living through the second wave of Covid-19. The idea for this book began a year ago, in September of 2019. What a year. The world is a very different place; things we took for granted have changed for the foreseeable future. Perhaps forever. We are adapting to a "new normal." This pandemic has devastated many people's lives, and I certainly empathize with their pain and loss. For some, it has cost them their lives; for others, it has cost them their livelihood; and for many, it creates fear of what the future holds—paralyzing fear preventing positive actions from being taken to secure a desirable future. This group of society binge-watch the media, scroll through social media, and perpetuate the spread of fearmongering.

For some, this time has provided the opportunity to reflect, recharge, and reset. It's how they choose to see the situation. It's not that their lives aren't affected, but it is how they have dealt with it. For me, the past year has been a period of growth. I've been working on identifying and improving my weaknesses. In all areas of my life. Physical, mental and spiritual. I have witnessed many friends and colleagues hide, become unfit, binge on Netflix and allow themselves to wallow in negativity. No thank you.

Prior to the pandemic, I had signed up for an ultra-marathon race slated for mid-September 2020. Like many other things, it was canceled, but I still put in the training. At 6'1" and a lean 200 pounds I do not possess the ideal physique of an endurance runner. So, I started researching ultra-endurance athletes and came across Rich Roll. Author, ultra-endurance athlete, entrepreneur, and so much more. I read his book *Finding Ultra*, which I highly recommend.

The first change that I made was my fueling. I do not diet and exercise; I eat and train.

I have tried various food plans, from the Keto diet to the Zone diet, Paleo, high carb low-fat diets, and a mix of others. I do not endorse or discount any of them. I have experienced an increase in my energy levels this past year. I feel better, sleep better, my endurance has improved, and I've shed 10 pounds of body fat. How? I have become a vegan. From the guy that used to eat a double cheeseburger with bacon two to three times a week, I am the first to be shocked. I would have likely laughed had you told me a year ago I would be consuming a plant-based diet. But I am a firm believer in trying something for myself before judging it. I encourage you to do the same.

For the past five years, health and fitness have become my way of life. I am committed wholeheartedly to doing the work. Training five days a week and consciously aligning mind, body, and spirit. Excuses are not an option. If the gyms are closed, I train outdoors. If there are no barbells, I use a kettlebell, sandbags, rocks, logs, and my own body weight. I run, ruck and swim. Fitness doesn't take holidays or stop for a pandemic.

My clients feel the same way and have continued training without missing a beat. We follow Covid protocols and maintain a safety-first regime. We believe that the way to beat illness is to stay healthy. What we do today will determine our quality of life tomorrow.

We are still learning about Covid-19, but we know that like many diseases, if you are overweight, above a certain age, live a sedentary lifestyle and don't make an effort to change, you are at a much higher risk of suffering life-threatening consequences.

So what are you going to do now? Are you going to get off the couch and take responsibility for your future? Are you going to be there for your grandkids? Are you going to enjoy retirement feeling fit? Don't let your present situation dictate your future. Don't let an excuse get in the way of taking immediate action. When the little voice in your head says you can't, Do it Anyway!

I wish you great success, the type that does not come at the cost of your health and happiness. And if I can help you reach your goals just reach out and let me know.

– Scott Harlow
September 2020

ACKNOWLEDGEMENTS

Mom and Dad for the freedom to pursue my dreams. For allowing me to learn from my failures, and for unconditional love and support.

Payton, for bringing our beautiful children into the world.

Liam, Marin, and Maddy. The most amazing kids a dad could wish for.

Jim and Joanne. For always being there for me.

Coach Mark Divine for the life changing Kokoro moment. I will forever be in your debt.

Jason McCarthy, CEO at GORUCK for hosting Selection, the hardest endurance event on the planet, and to the cadre that force us to uphold the special forces standards. I learned so much from you and look forward to learning more in the future.

Coach Cam Birtwell of Crossfit VicCity. I could not have completed Kokoro 44 without you.

Coach Brad Macleod of SEALGRINDER PT for helping me take my fitness to a level that I never believed possible.

To Nathan Isbister for inspiring me to enroll in Kokoro 51 and for being a great friend and training partner.

Special thanks to Raul Rodriguez, Jim Steg, and Rick Steele, and the rest of my Kokoro teammates for teaching me how to be a better team player and leader.

Last but certainly not least Aaron Bethune. Publisher and co-writer of this book. For his vision, knowledge, and creativity.

ABOUT THE AUTHOR

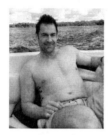 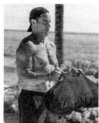

Scott Harlow is an ultra-endurance athlete, fitness coach, actor, dad, and sober alcoholic.

Having turned his health around at almost fifty and completing his first ultra-endurance event at fifty-one, Scott aspires to help others over forty take control of their health and fitness.

Breaking through his own perceived physical and mental limits, he is committed to helping others learn, grow, and change their situations to improve their quality of life.

At the core of his beliefs is his Do It Anyway mentality.

Scott lives in Victoria, British Columbia, on Vancouver Island, where he trains people from around the world.

For free sample workouts, contact the author at scott@scottharlow.ca